# Prosthetics and Orthotics

*Edited by Mokhtar Arazpour*

Published in London, United Kingdom

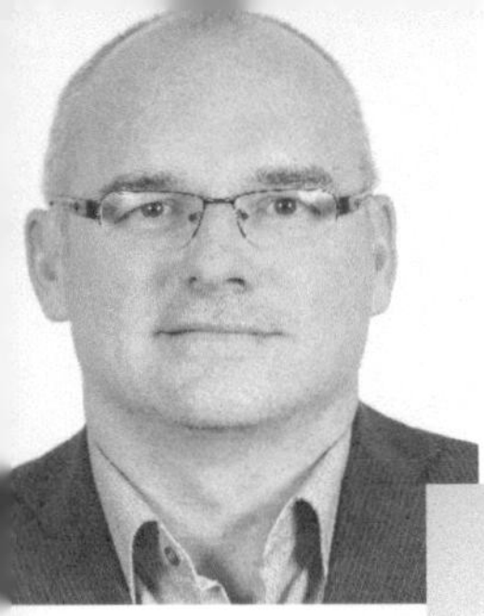
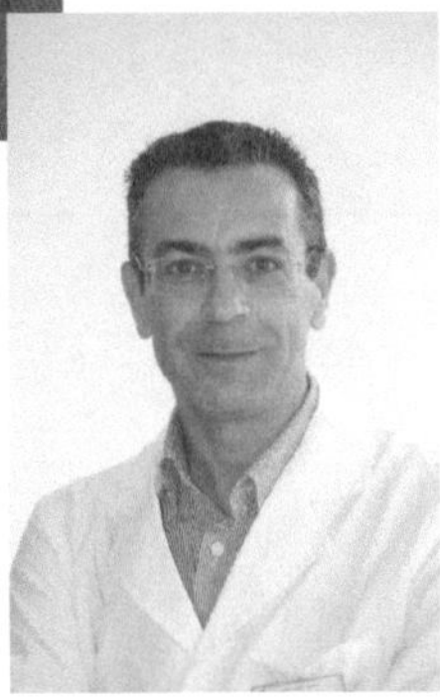
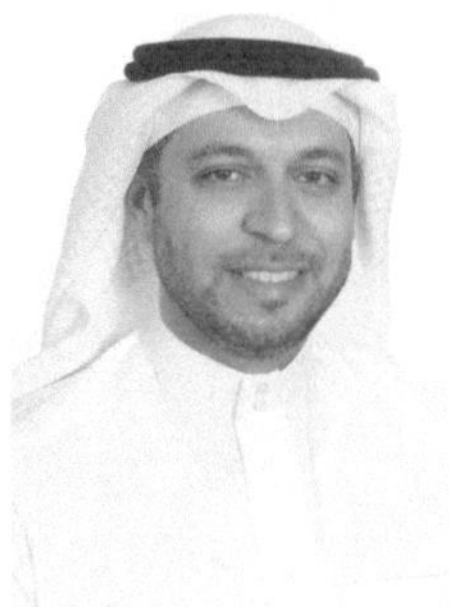
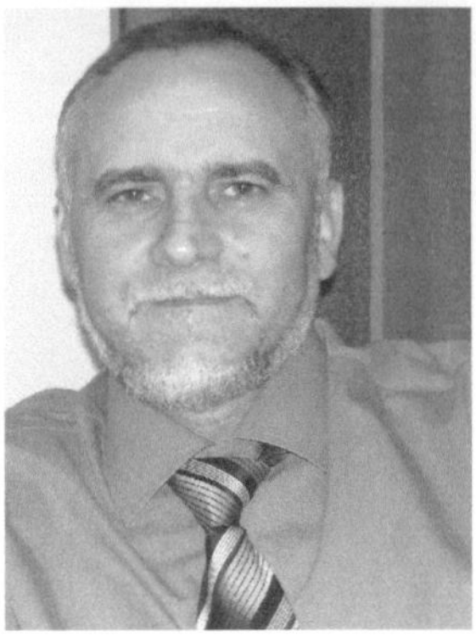
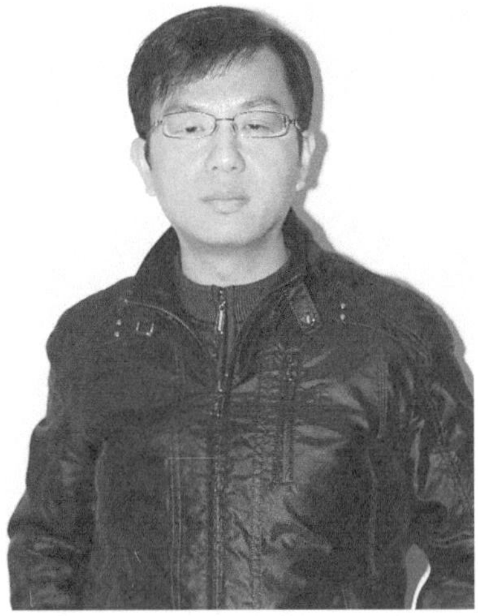
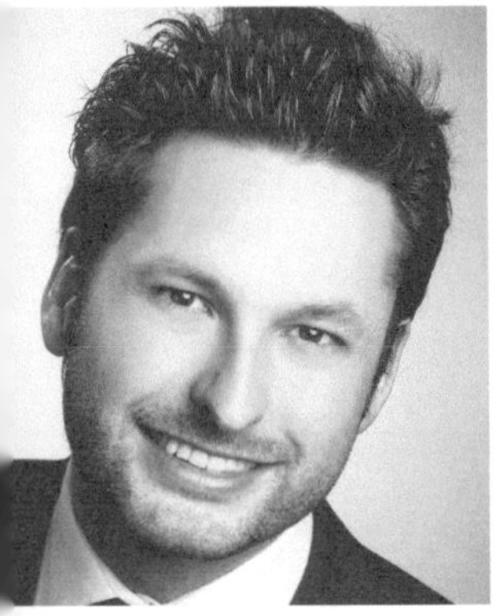
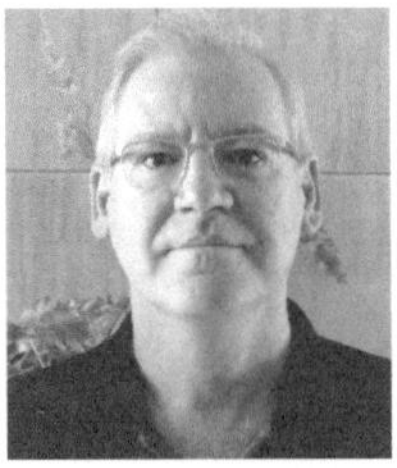

IntechOpen

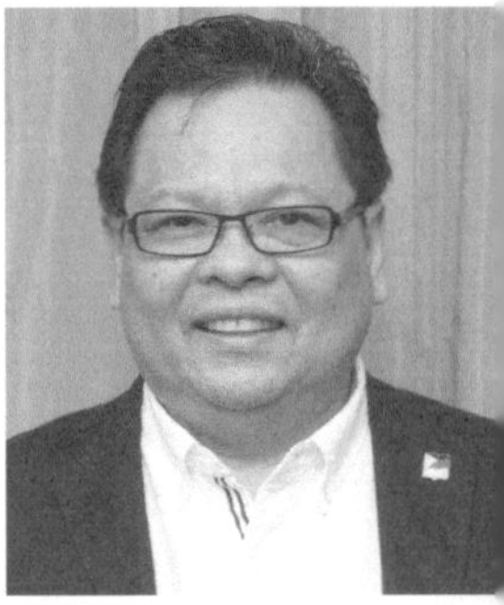
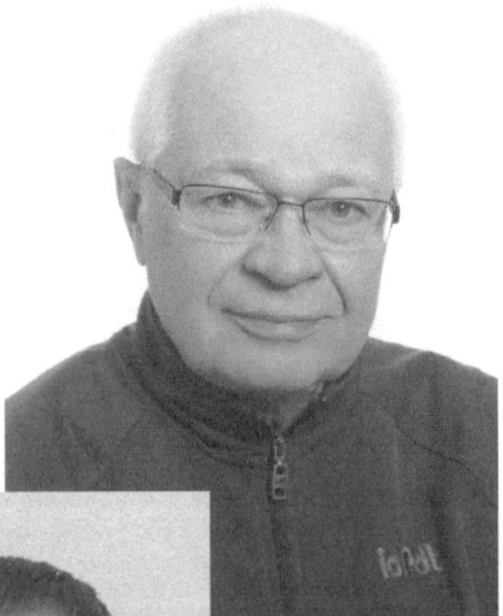
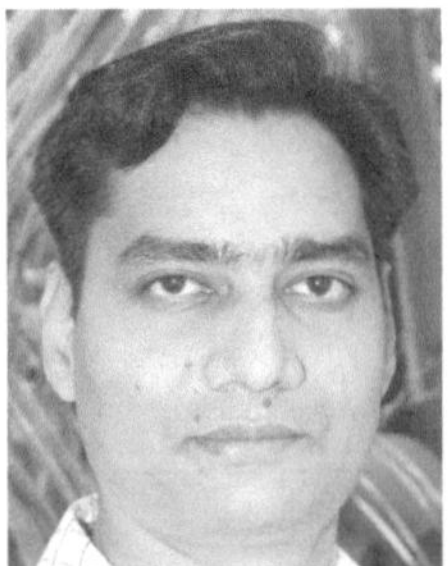
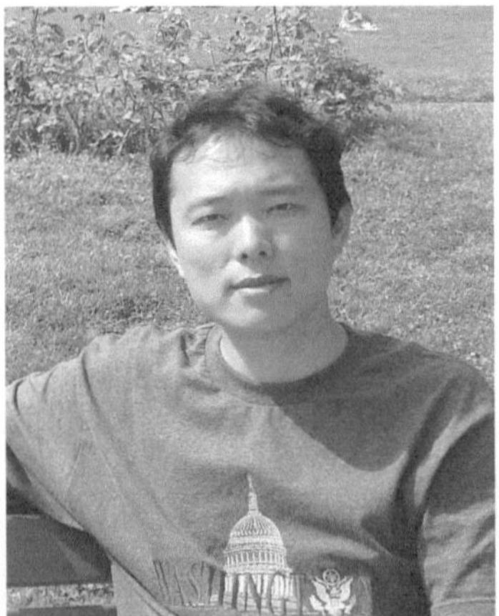
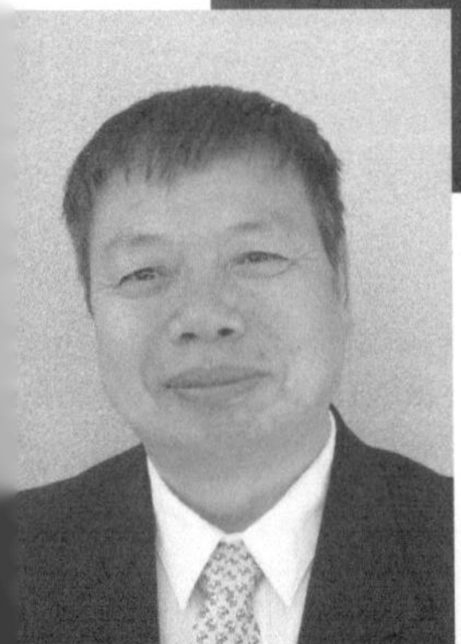
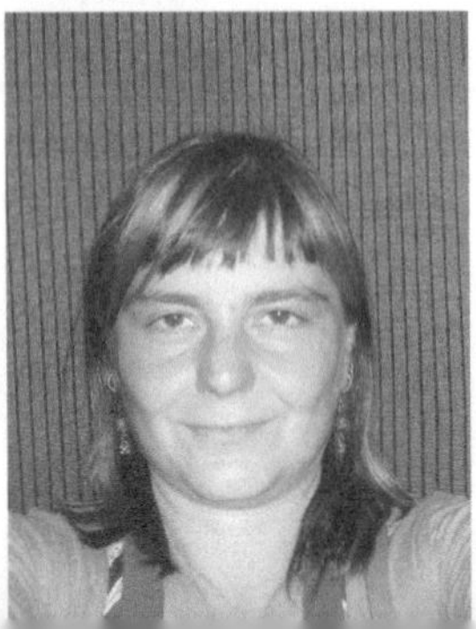

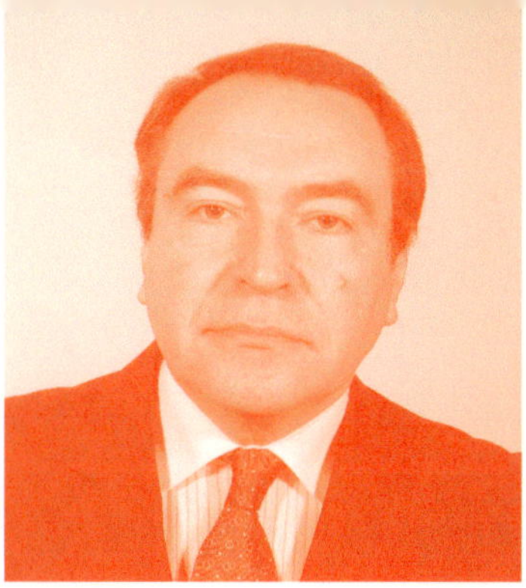

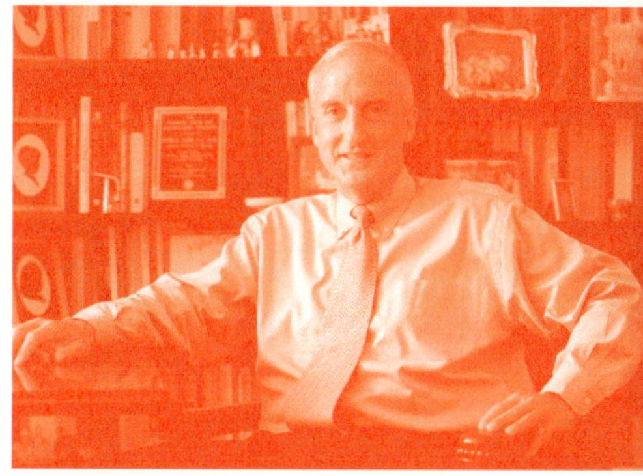

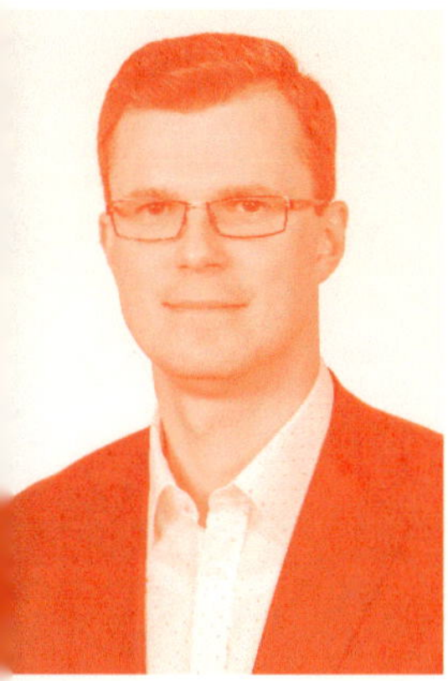

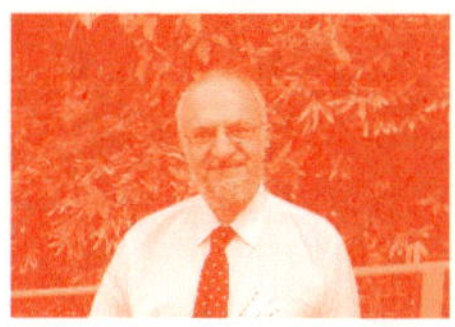

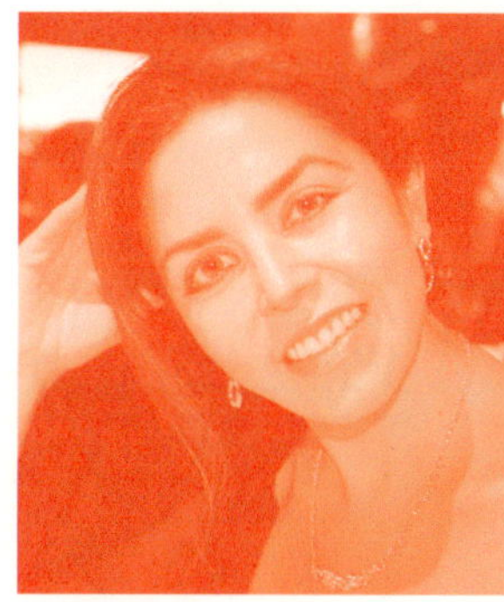

*Supporting open minds since 2005*

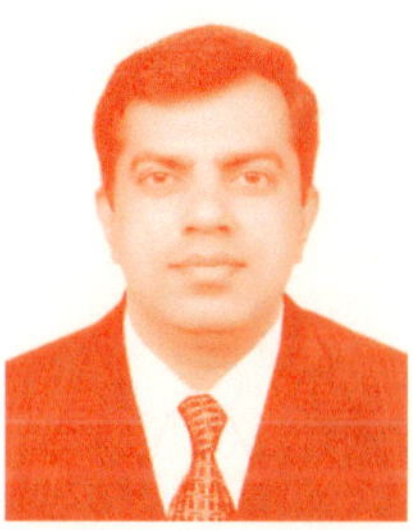

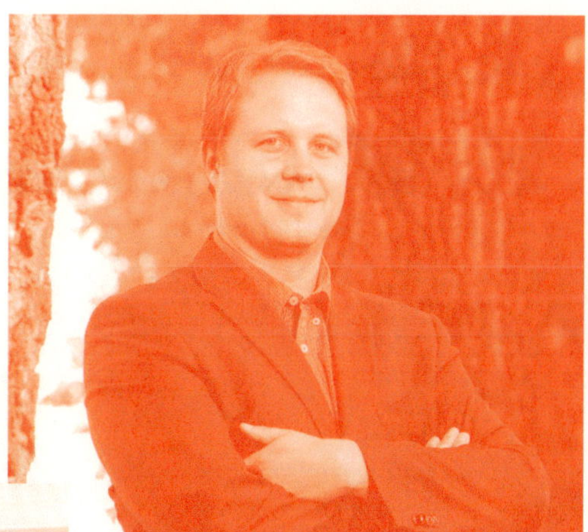

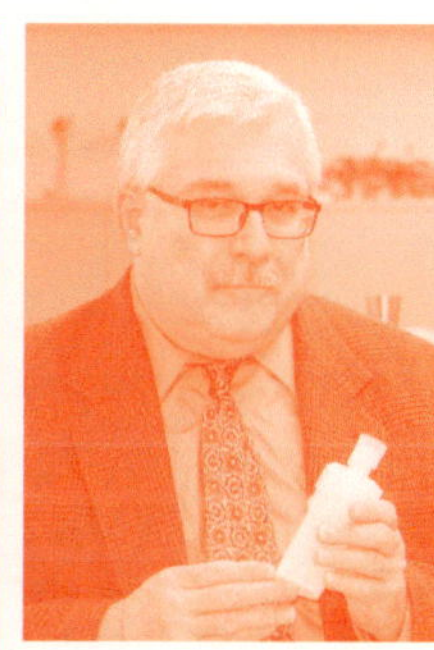

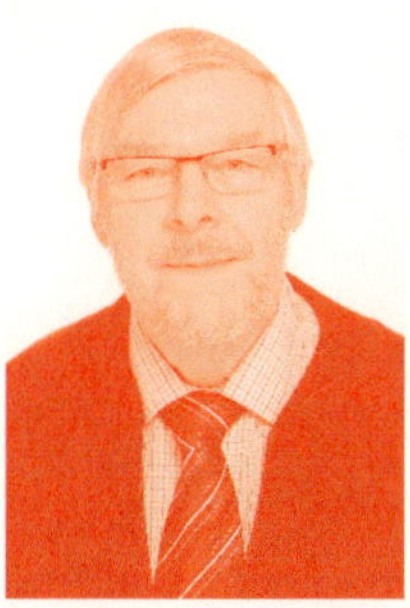

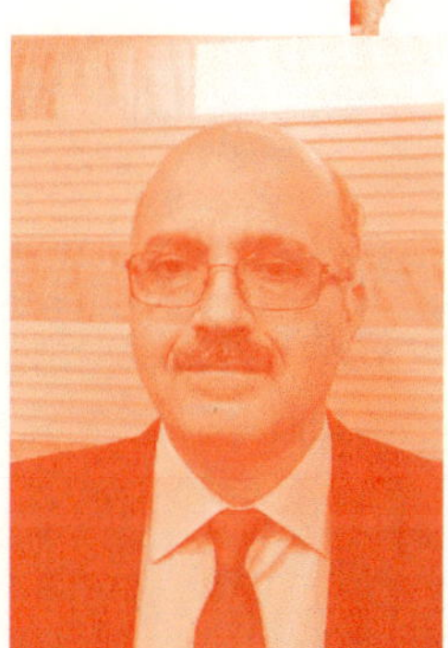

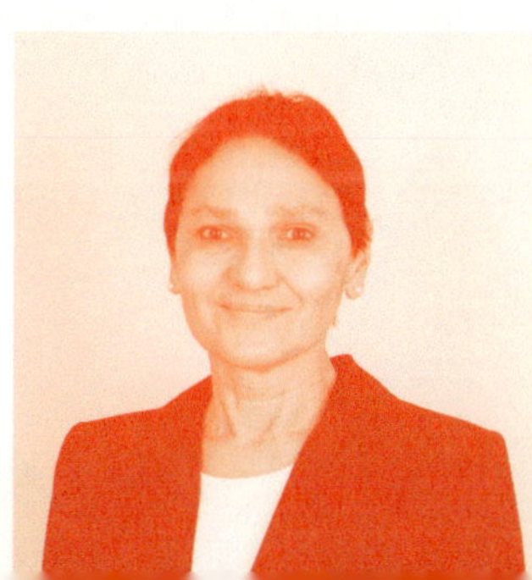

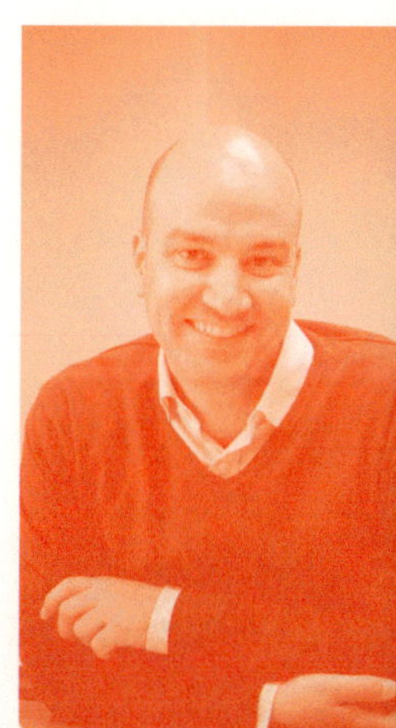

Prosthetics and Orthotics
http://dx.doi.org/10.5772/intechopen.90812
Edited by Mokhtar Arazpour

Contributors
Benjamin Dourthe, Judith Osterloh, Vinzenz Von Tscharner, Sandro Nigg, Benno M. Nigg, Harish Kumar Kumar Banga, Parveen Kalra, Rajendra.M Belokar, Rajesh Kumar, Branko Štefanovič, Mária Danko, Monika Michalíková, Lucia Bednarčíková, Viktória Rajťúková, Teodor Tóth, Marianna Trebuňová, Radovan Hudak, Jozef Zivcak, P. Senthil Selvam, M. Sandhiya, K. Chandrasekaran, S. Karthikeyan, D. Hepzibah Rubella, Ashish Castellino, Mohan Kameswaran, Akshay Kumar, Vinita, Mokhtar Arazpour, Cristina Gonzalez-Martin, Maria Teresa Garcia-Rodriguez, Sonia Pertega-Diaz, Rocio Seijo-Bestilleiro



First published in London, United Kingdom, 2021 by IntechOpen
IntechOpen is the global imprint of INTECHOPEN LIMITED, registered in England and Wales, registration number: 11086078, 5 Princes Gate Court, London, SW7 2QJ, United Kingdom
Printed in Croatia

British Library Cataloguing-in-Publication Data
A catalogue record for this book is available from the British Library

Additional hard and PDF copies can be obtained from orders@intechopen.com

Prosthetics and Orthotics
Edited by Mokhtar Arazpour
p. cm.
Print ISBN 978-1-83962-900-6
Online ISBN 978-1-83962-901-3
eBook (PDF) ISBN 978-1-83962-905-1

# Meet the editor

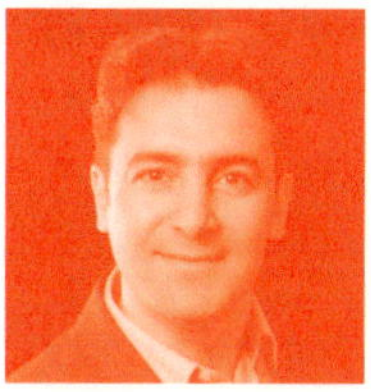

Dr. Mokhtar Arazpour is an associate professor in the Department of Orthotics and Prosthetics, University of Social Welfare and Rehabilitation Sciences (USWR), Tehran, Iran, where he also obtained his BS, MSc, and Ph.D. in Orthotics and Prosthetics. The title of his Ph.D. thesis is "Design, Construction, and Evaluation of the New Powered Gait Orthosis for Walking in Spinal Cord Injury Patients." Dr. Arazpour's research interests include lower-limb orthotics, osteoarthritis of knee and hand joints, design and construction of new lower limb orthosis, and walking analysis.

# Contents

# Preface

In recent years, many changes have taken place in the field of rehabilitation of people who need prostheses and orthoses. Advancement of technology, significant progress in computer components and robotics, and the development of new materials have enabled many people in need to return to useful and practical life. Subjects who have lost their limbs or parts of their limbs can now continue to work and perform activities of daily living.

In line with these changes, the expectations of prosthetic and orthodontic therapists have also changed dramatically. Therapists in this field are currently trained in graduate school and are expected to research, develop, implement, or monitor the application of complex interventions. This book provides information for effective clinical decision-making for those working with people who need prosthetics and orthoses. It is also designed to assist prosthetists and orthotists to acquire the knowledge and skills necessary for effective membership in the physical therapy team.

The book is divided into two parts. The first part covers the field of prosthetics and the second part covers the field of orthotics. Each part discusses construction methods, applications, and effects of prosthetic and orthotic devices.

This book is a resource for all physicians to use to increase their ability to provide the most up-to-date care for all people in need of prostheses or orthoses.

**Mokhtar Arazpour**
University of Social Welfare and Rehabilitation Sciences,
Iran

Section 1

# Prosthetics

Chapter 1

# Introductory Chapter: Technology and Orthotics and Prosthetics

*Mokhtar Arazpour*

## 1. Introduction

In recent years, the use of technology has seen significant growth in the design and manufacture of advanced and intelligent orthoses and prostheses. Progress has been made in 4 areas in orthosis and prosthetics.

1) Material 2) Fabrication approach 3) Intelligent joints for orthoses 4) Intelligent joint in prostheses.

This has been accompanied by increasing growth in the materials used to make orthoses and prostheses. Activities of subject, the weight of the user are two important issues in used materials in fabrication of orthoses and prostheses for each subject. Flexible polymers, Carbon fiber, Kevlar and titanium are materials that were used to provide comfort and the strength and durability of the fabricated devices [1].

Computer-aided design/computer-aided manufacturing (CAD/CAM) technology is new manner to design and fabricate each type of orthoses and prostheses [2]. Scanning done by laser or hand held wand to provide measurement of limb. Based on this information the size and shape of limbs is given to prosthetist-orthotist to design and fabricate the mentioned orthoses and prostheses for the subject by computer [3].

Subjects with poliomyelitis, incomplete spinal cord injury and quadriceps weakness who have not knee stabilization during walking used devices with locked knee joints [4]. Walking with this condition provided high energy consumption and fatigue. Stance control knee joints are new generation of orthoses that developed in recent years in the world by many different companies [5]. Some of this type of joints is intelligent and smart that provided stability in stance phase and free swing during walking [6].

Intelligent prostheses can now be fabricated for the subjects with amputation [7]. This type of prosthesis in the lower limb permits the knee joint to sense alternation in position, speed and force, enabling subjects with amputations to walk down stairs and hills with confidence [8]. There were many developments in the prosthetic feet for running and other sport conditions. In the upper limbs prostheses, electrically powered units were used. This type of prosthesis can detect myoelectric signals provided by muscles to control the prosthesis [9].

Development in provided different orthoses and prostheses with advanced technology cause the prosthetist/orthotist is well trained and educated to construct devices based on the subject needs of each patient and to develop appropriate suggestions.

**Author details**

Mokhtar Arazpour
University of Social Welfare and Rehabilitation Sciences, Tehran, Iran

*Address all correspondence to: m.arazpour@yahoo.com

## References

[1] Wong MS, Beygi BH, Zheng Y. Materials for exoskeletal orthotic and prosthetic systems. Encyclopedia of Biomedical Engineering: Elsevier; 2018. p. 352-67.

[2] Supan TJ. Principles of fabrication. Atlas of Orthoses and Assistive Devices: Elsevier; 2019. p. 42-8. e1.

[3] Banga HK, Kalra P, Belokar RM, Kumar R. Design and Fabrication of Prosthetic and Orthotic Product by 3D Printing. Orthotics and Prosthetics: IntechOpen; 2020.

[4] Moreno JC, Brunetti F, Rocon E, Pons JL. Immediate effects of a controllable knee ankle foot orthosis for functional compensation of gait in patients with proximal leg weakness. Medical & biological engineering & computing. 2008;46(1):43-53.

[5] Del-Ama AJ, Koutsou AD, Moreno JC, De-Los-Reyes A, Gil-Agudo Á, Pons JL. Review of hybrid exoskeletons to restore gait following spinal cord injury. Journal of Rehabilitation Research & Development. 2012;49(4).

[6] Fatone S. A review of the literature pertaining to KAFOs and HKAFOs for ambulation. JPO: Journal of Prosthetics and Orthotics. 2006;18(7):P137-P68.

[7] Cochrane H, Orsi K, Reilly P. Lower limb amputation Part 3: Prosthetics-a 10 year literature review. Prosthetics and orthotics international. 2001;25(1):21-8.

[8] Laferrier JZ, Gailey R. Advances in lower-limb prosthetic technology. Physical Medicine and Rehabilitation Clinics. 2010;21(1):87-110.

[9] Herrmann S, Attenberger A, Buchenrieder K, editors. Prostheses control with combined near-infrared and myoelectric signals. International Conference on Computer Aided Systems Theory; 2011: Springer.

Chapter 2

# Prosthetics for Lower Limb Amputation

*P. Senthil Selvam, M. Sandhiya, K. Chandrasekaran, D. Hepzibah Rubella and S. Karthikeyan*

## Abstract

The Chapter will include a brief note on Amputation, Particularly Lower Limb Amputation (LLA), Levels and Causes of LLA. Importance of Prosthetics for LLA are explained in detail. The types of Prosthesis, Application (Donning & Doffing) of prosthesis are included in this chapter. Diagrammatic representation of the prosthesis are added too. Bio mechanical component is explained in detail within this chapter. The advantages and disadvantages of each and every Lower limb Prosthesis are clearly mentioned. Moreover, the Gait analysis & Training after the application of prosthesis are discussed. The reader will get a complete picture of Prosthetics for Lower limb Amputation by going through this chapter for lower limb prosthesis.

**Keywords:** lower limb prosthesis, donning & doffing, advantages & disadvantages of prosthesis, materials used for prosthesis, types of prosthesis

## 1. Introduction

This chapter is written to give information about the basic knowledge about the prosthesis, its types, its application and its advantages. The readers can understand the concept of Prosthesis with respect to biomechanical principles and how the Amputee can adapt himself to the usage of prosthesis with simple explanation. Hence, the chapter gives a overview about the lower limb prosthesis with illustrated pictures for better understanding.

Prosthetics are otherwise known as artificial limbs. They are the device used to replace a missing limb, either upper limb or lower limb. Thereby, the prosthesis are used by a amputee. The amputee by wearing this device, can able to stand walks, maintain balance and regain erect posture. The science of creating artificial body parts is called prosthetics. This prosthesis is designed and manufactured by prosthetist. He also fits the artificial limbs (prosthesis) for people with disabilities especially amputees.

## 2. Lower limb prostheses

Prostheses is most commonly prescriped for lower limb amputation. Amputation is defined as the removal of the limb through a part of the bone [1] the lower limb amputation is the most common amputation nearly 85 percent of all amputations. The function of lower limb is weight bearing and locomotion. Lower limb prostheses is used to provide an individual who has an amputated limb with the opportunity to perform functional tasks, particularly ambulation (walking) which may not be possible without the limb.

## 3. Types of lower limb prostheses

The types of prostheses (**Figure 1**) is determined by an extend of the level of amputation (**Figure 2**). The lower limb amputation are performed at different levels based on that the prostheses are developed. The types of prostheses are

1. Hemipelvectomy prostheses – for hemipelvectomy surgeries
2. Hip disarticulation prostheses – for hip disarticulation
3. Above knee prostheses – Transfemoral/Above knee amputation.
4. Below knee prostheses - Transtibial/below knee amputation. The prosthetic socket encases the residual limb , and is often classified as either "Patellar tendon bearing" - dispersing weight distribution onto several pressure tolerance areas including patellar tendon or "Total surface bearing" creating more equal weight distribution throughout the entire socket.
5. Symes prostheses - Symes amputation/Ankle disarticulation [1]

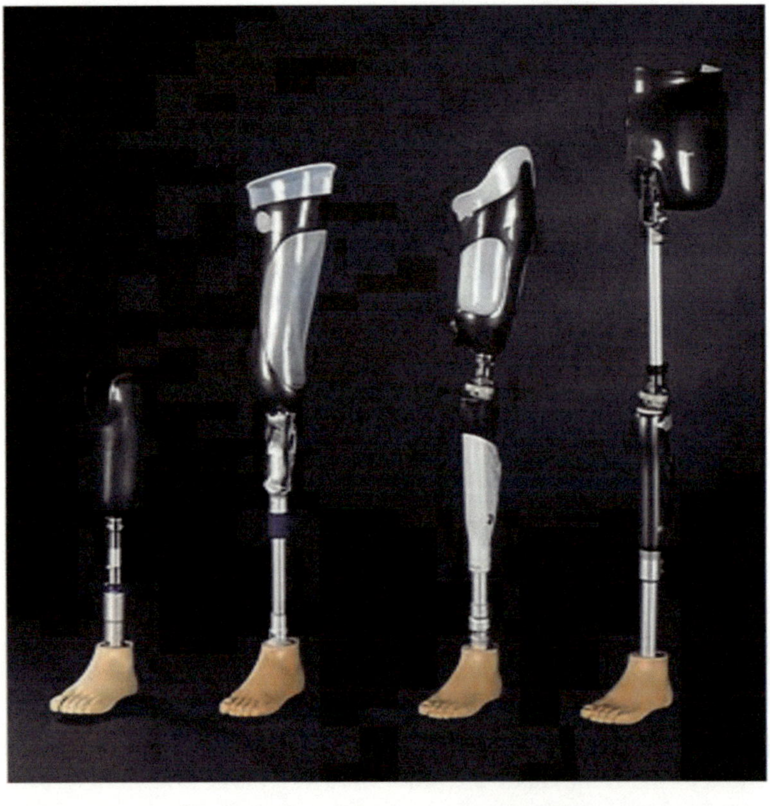

**Figure 1.**
*Types of Prostheses.*

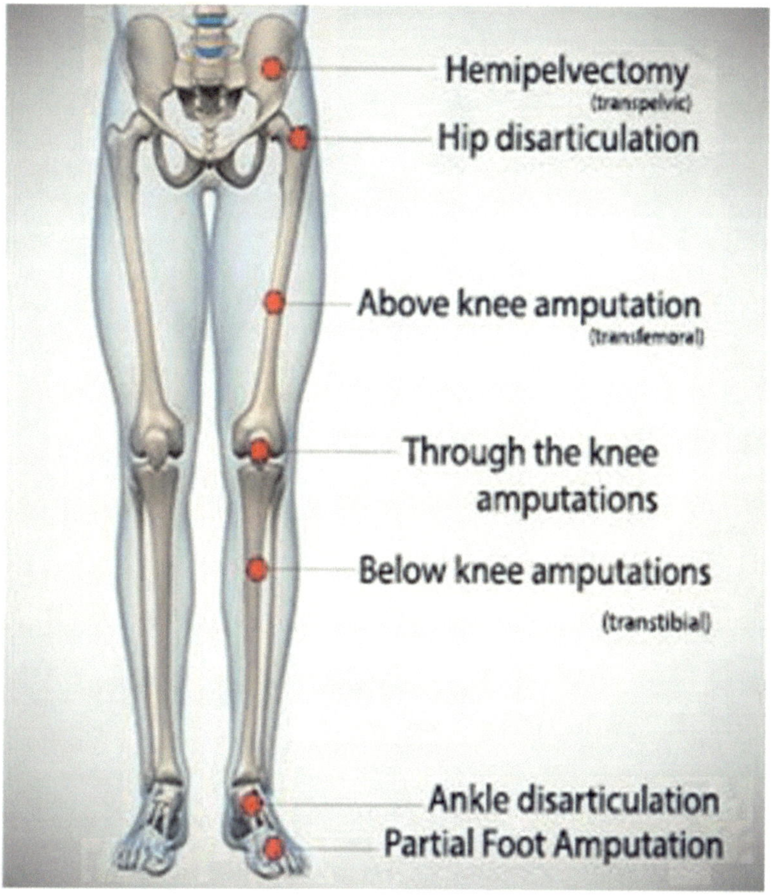


**Figure 2.**
*Levels of amputation.*

## 4. Prosthetic construction design

The prosthetics are designed into two types

i. Endoskeletal prostheses

ii. Exoskeletal prostheses

### 4.1 Endoskeletal prostheses

Endoskeletal prostheses (**Figure 3**) is a type of prostheses in which the supporting structure is internal it is also called as modular prostheses, it is most commonly used type of prostheses. The endoskeletal prostheses use the human skeleton as the model it has the tube frame provides the weight bearing function and a foam cover gives the prostheses it's near natural appearance [2]. A tube frame is a central part it is called as pylon. The pylon is constructed from Aluminium, Titanium or Stainless steel, it connect proximally socket and distally prosthetic foot. The endoskeletal prostheses includes the joint components to suit the need of the individual amputee.

Advantages of endoskeletal prostheses are

- Changes may be done at any point of time

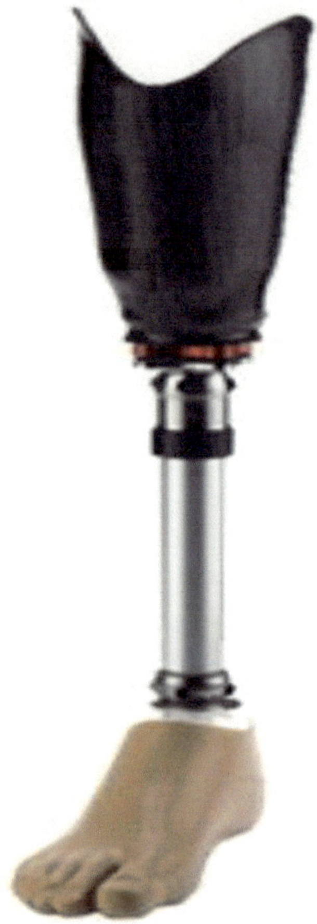

**Figure 3.**
*Endoskeletal prostheses.*

- Light weight and comfortable for weight bearing
- Cosmetically acceptable and it gives the appearance of near to normal
- Suitable for all levels of amputation
- It gives adequate adjustment and good dynamic alignment.

Disadvantages

- Less resistant to external wear
- The foam cover is not last for a longer period and needs to be changed often.

### 4.2 Exoskeletal prostheses

The exoskeletal prostheses (**Figure 4**) is a type of prostheses in which the supporting structure are on outside. It is also called as conventional or crustacean prostheses. The exoskeletal prostheses has a rigid outer shell as a supporting structure it provides shape and weight bearing function. The weight is beared through

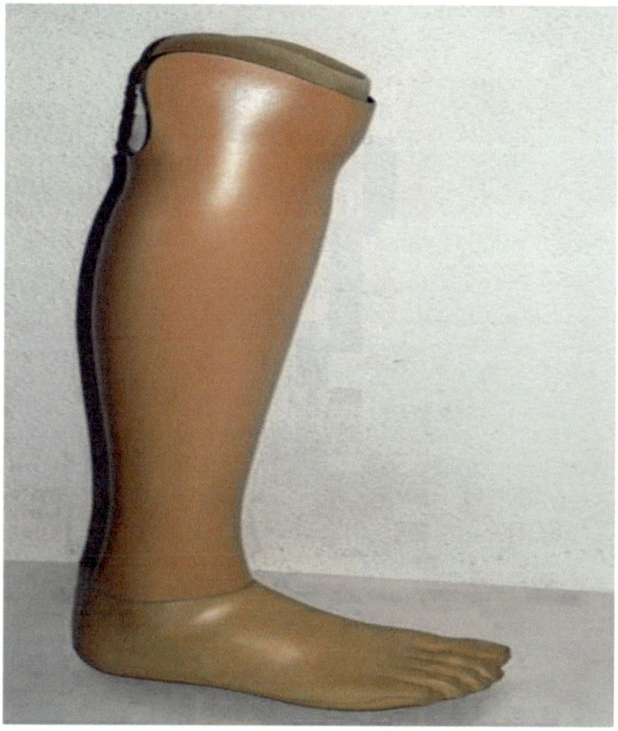

**Figure 4.**
*Exoskeletal prostheses.*

the outer shell. It is constructed of wood, or rigid polyurethane covered with a rigid plastic lamination [3].

Advantages of exoskeletal prostheses are

- Lasted for a longer period
- More resistant to external wear
- Cost effective

Disadvantages are

- Heavy & uncomfortable for use
- Fabrication time is longer
- Alignment cannot be changed & couldn't be adjusted
- Not suitable for through knee amputation.

## 5. Components of lower limb prostheses

The lower limb prostheses has the following components (**Figure 5**)

1. Socket : Is the most important part it is the connection between the stump and the prosthesis. It protects the stump and transmits forces. Contoured sockets

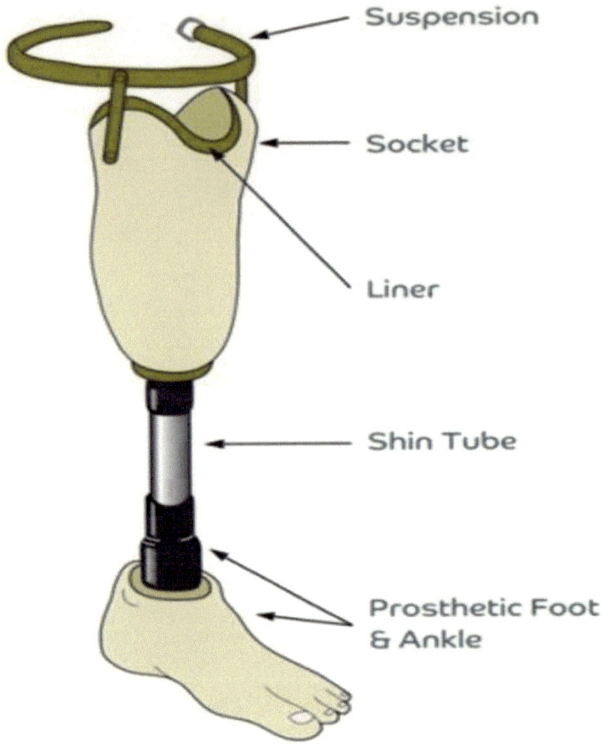


**Figure 5.**
*Components of lower limb prostheses.*

fit closer to bone, muscle, soft tissue. It provide support. It can be made of thermoplastic or metal.

2. Suspension : This holds the artificial limb on to stump. Eg. Sleeve, belt, straps, cuffs, suction prostheses.

3. Liner : This is a removable inner socket made of flexible material.

4. Pylon or Shank : This lies between the socket and the prosthetic foot. It is made of strong and lightweight material such as Carbon fibre, Aluminium & Titanium.

5. Prosthetic foot & ankle : Designed to provide support during standing/walking and shock absorption.

## 6. Description of lower limb prostheses

### 6.1 Design of prostheses

The prostheses required a high level of customization and represents the interface with the human body or parts of it, the artificial prostheses that have to be designed according to the shape of the specific anatomical area. Considerations taken into account when designing prostheses are basic structure of a lower limb prostheses, materials, weight and mass considerations, power requirements, biomechanics, and tradeoffs in motion and stability.

#### *6.1.1 Temporary prostheses*

The temporary prostheses is also called as preparatory prostheses. Temporary prostheses are used for early rehabilitation purpose to speeds the recovery process and it ease the transition into a definitive prostheses. The advantage of the temporary prostheses is it fastened the mobility of the amputee postoperatively, prevents the complications of prolonged bed rest and it promote early discharge from the hospital. It's applied within few days after surgery and limited early gait training is given.

Indications are

- Applied for early rehabilitation
- Unhealed residual limb like Burns, Skin grafts, Open wounds, Infection.
- Dermatological condition
- Painful residual limb
- Fracture healing process

#### *6.1.2 Permanent prostheses*

The permanent prosthesis is also called as definitive prostheses. It is applied when the surgical wound is completely healed and the residual limb become shrinken and shaped. The permanent prostheses is changed when the prostheses become excess wear and the atrophy of the residual limb. The permanent prostheses are should be proper fit there by the patient will get proper weight bearing & movement.

#### *6.1.3 Special-use prostheses*

The prostheses are specifically designed for certain number of patients will require special-use prostheses and it is designed specifically for sports activities such as running, swimming, or skiing. Special-use prostheses can be valuable to the amputee who wishes to expand his activities and participate in a full range of sports and recreation.

### 6.2 Materials used

The various materials are used to design the prostheses, the materials should be strong enough, light weight, resistant to thermal conditions, longer durability and biocompatible it should not cause allergic reactions to the body. The materials are

1. Metals: Titanium, Aluminium and stainless steel. The metals are used both in exo & endoskeletal prostheses e.g Socket, Pylon.
2. Plastic: Socket is made of plastic, the thermoplastic materials like polypropylene, polyethylene, polyurethane, acrylic are commonly used. The thermosetting plastic also used for laminated sockets in which the resin is combined with the reinforcing materials like glass fibre, nylon,carban fibre.
3. Wood: Is used in lowerlimb prostheses for foot assembly e.g SACH foot Solid-ankle, cushion-heel (SACH) feet have an interior hardwood heel that provides structural strength to the foot. This heel is bolted to the rest of the prosthesis.

4. Leather: Is used for suspension straps, socket linings.

5. Rubber: The foot in the prostheses made by vulganised rubber

6. Fabric/cotton: Socks is made of cotton. Socks are used as an interface between residual limb & socket and it provides comfort & prevent friction between the residual limb and socket.

7. Fiber reinforcement: Two basic types of high-strength fiber reinforcements are used in prosthetics are glass and carbon. Carbon fibers are more expensive than fiberglass but have superior strength and stiffness. Carbon fibers are generally set in epoxy and can provide a material with a stiffness. In addition to this high strength-to-weight ratio, carbon fiber composites have a fatigue resistance. Prefabricated carbon fiber prosthetic components such as pylon tubes, knee joints, and connectors can significantly reduce the weight of the prosthesis while increasing its strength.

### 6.3 Function of prostheses

1. To substitute for a lost limb

2. To restore function of Amputee

3. Comfortable ambulation

4. Reduce expenditure of energy

5. Minimizing the shift of the center of gravity of the body during gait.

### 6.4 Advantages of prostheses

Loss of limb not only causes physical handicap but also leads to Social, Psychological and economic effects on the individual and family. This loss can be overcome to a greater extent by the application of artificial limb which restores the function as well as total body image.

### 6.5 Disadvantages of prostheses

1. Choke syndrome - caused by obstructed venous outflow due to tight socket leads to red, indurated skin with orange-peel appearance, venous stasis ulcers.

2. Skin problems:

    - Contact dermatitis most commonly caused by liner, socks, and suspension mechanism

    - Cysts

    - Hyperhydrosis

3. Erythema, skin damage – due to shear forces and improperly fit of prostheses.

4. Painful residual limb – due to pressure in the bony prominence.

## 7. Above knee amputation

Above Knee Amputation (AK Amputation) is Removing the Three Fourth Of The Leg from the body by cutting through femoral muscle and bone. The optimum length of the residual bone is approximately 7.5 – 10cm proximal to the superior border of the patella. With a AK amputation the distal attachments of the femoral muscles are lost, in order to preserve their length and functions myodesis may be performed.

### 7.1 Indications

Trauma
Malignant Tumors
Diabetic Gangrene
Infections
Peripheral Artery Disease
Burns

### 7.2 Above knee prosthesis

An above knee prosthesis also known as transfemoral prosthesis. It is custom made for the person who have undergone above knee amputation.

### 7.3 Components of above knee prosthetics

1. Suspension

2. Cosmesis

3. Socket

4. Knee Joint

5. Shank

6. Foot Ankle Unit

#### *7.3.1 Suspension*

Suspension is the part which holds the residual limb into the Socket. Rigid belts or straps can be used as primary suspension which is suspended around the pelvis. This helps the socket on and prevent it from falling off during swing phase. A good suspension will enhance the control of prosthesis, improve energy transfer and decrease discomfort or difficulty during walking. The disadvantages of suspension includes causes pressure around the pelvis, needs good strength and dexterity of hand, moves when sitting, can cause bruising and irritation.

#### *7.3.2 Cosmesis*

It is the cosmetic cover that gives a shape and apprearence to the artificial limb. Most of the aritificial limbs are covered with a continous foamtube. This foam tube is made to match with the remaining limb as close as possible. Later it is covered with stockings.

*7.3.3 Socket*

The socket for an above knee amputee has two basic categories.

a. ISCHIAL CONTAINMENT SOCKETS: This type of socket have a rigid frame with a flexible inner socket, which holds the pelvis inside the socket.

b. QUADRILATERAL SOCKET: This type of socket provides a shelf for the pelvis to sit on the brim of the socket.

*7.3.4 Knee joint*

This part is designed to stabilise the individual during standing and walking by transmitting weight throught he prosthesis.it is of two types

a. A SINGLE AXIS: This type enables the individual to bent and straight knee joint in single direction.

b. POLYCENTRIC KNEE: This type allows knee to bend in different directions. this helps in walking on uneven surfaces.

*7.3.5 SHANK*

This part connects the foot and ankle with the socket. There are two types of shanks.

a. Endoskeletal design: This is lightweighted soft foam gives appearance of skin . It is easily adjustable and compatible with advance technology. But the disadvantage is foam cover is fragile and can be damaged.

b. Exoskeletal design: This type has rigid and durable shell made up of laminated material. This is more durable than endoskeleton .It the ability to transfer weight throught the entire design.

*7.3.6 Foot ankle unit*

This is the vital part prosthetics to provide support while the individual stands on the prosthesis. The following are the various designs of prosthetic feet.

a. SACH (SOLID ANKLE CUSHION HEEL). It provides a single motion on the joint. This is relatively lightweighted, durable and less expessive.

b. SINGLE AXIS FOOT. This provides up and down movement enhancing knee stability.

c. MULTIAXIS FOOT. This provides increased mobility at the ankle, which helps stabilize the individual on uneven surfaces.

d. DYNAMIC RESPONSE FOOT. This type is more preferable for the individual who can vary in walking speed, change directions quickly and for long distances.it provides a normal range of motion and more symmetric gait [4].

### 7.4 Application of prosthesis

#### *7.4.1 Donning the prosthesis*

STEP 1- Check for any signs of skin breakdown in residual limb
STEP 2- Open areas should be cleaned and covered with proper gauze bandage
STEP 3- Put on adequate number of socks to fit the residual limb into socket too loose and too tight socks should be avoided.
STEP 4- Clear the wrinkles on the sock to smoothen the surface
STEP 5-Bend the prosthesis knee to 90 degree with the foot flat
STEP 6- Slide the residual limb into the socket and fasten the suspension system loosely.
STEP 7- Stand up holding a stable surface like walker or table
STEP 8- Bring the prosthesis under the hip joint and straighten the prosthenic knee completely
STEP 9- Adjust the residual limb to fit into the socket and finally fasten the suspension system completely.

#### *7.4.2 Doffing the prosthesis*

STEP 1- Sit down and remove the suspension system
STEP 2- Remove the socket by slipping it off from the residual limb
STEP3- Check the limb for any signs of skin breakdown [5].

#### *7.4.3 Bilateral above knee amputation prosthesis*

It is also known as stubby prosthesis or stubbies. These are specially designed for individual with bilateral above knee amputation and those who are not eligible for full length prosthesis. They are custom fitted and are usually made up of standard sockets, no articulated knee joint with modified rocket bottom foot to prevent them from falling. Stubbies are foreshortened prostheses to bring down the center of gravity and thereby increase the stability. Suspension is achieved through the use of waist belts or pelvic straps. Advantages include stubbies are easy to apply and needs lesser energy expenditure from the patient. Disadvantages include sitting in a chair and stair climbing is difficult. Short canes and crutches are usually needed for the support. Cosmetically unaccepted because of the extreme reduction in height of the patient.

## 8. Below knee amputation

Below knee amputation (BK) also known as trastibial amputation. It is the surgical removal of foot , ankle and lower third of tibia and fibula. During BK Amputaion fibula is normally 2-3 cm shorter than the tibia to avoid pressure points.

### 8.1 Indications

Diabetic Foot
Traumatic Injury
Vascular Disease

Malignant Bone Tumors
Congenital Defects

## 8.2 Complications

Infections
Knee Contracture
Neuroma
Hetertopic Ossification
DVT
Pulmonary Embolism
Phantom Limb Pain

## 8.3 Below knee prosthesis

Below knee prosthesis also known as transtibialprosthesis. It is custom made for individual who have undergone bk amputation.

## 8.4 Components of below knee prosthesis

1. Suspension

2. Socket

3. Pylon

4. Ankle And Foot Unit

### *8.4.1 Suspension*

It is the part which holds the residual limb into the socket. Straps are used as support system to hold the socket into place. There are various types of suspension supracondylar cuff most common type, waist belt, cuff strap, thigh corset, vaccum suspension.

### *8.4.2 Socket*

This forms a connection between stump and prosthesis. It protects the stump and transmits the force. There are various types of sockets.

a. Conventional below knee socket

b. Patellar tendon bearing socket

c. Patellar tendon bearing and supracondylar suprapatellar socket

d. Bent knee socket

e. Slip socket

a. Conventional below knee socket: this is custom made for elderly people those with quadriceps weakening. It is fabricated with no pressure over distal tibia, fibula, head and tibial crest. It has disadvantage of skin irritation and stump chocking by edema.

b. Patellar tendon bearing socket: This is the commonly used socket. It is designed to load the weight in pressure bearing areas like patellor tendon and medial tibial flare. It has got a bar that is built in to patella tendon patella and tibial tubercle. Socket maintained at $5^0$ of knee flexion.

c. Patella tendon bearing supracondylar suprapatellar socket: It has anterior trim line to support suprapatellar region. It gives good suspension. It is very much useful for people with short stump and genu recurvatum.

d. Bent knee socket: It is designed for people with fixed flexion deformity. Upto $20^0$ of flexion can be accomodated.

e. Slip socket: It has two layers fine leather internally and wooden or plastic socket lines externally. It is also used for short stump.

#### *8.4.3 Pylon or shank*

It transfers the body weight from the socket to the foot.

Types of pylon

A. Exoskeletal

B. Endoskeletal

A. Exoskeletal: This is also known as conventinal type. Commonly designed with wood or plastic. The walls of the wooden components are resuced from inside. The exterior provides final shape and cannot be changed nce it is done. Disadvantages-Fabrication time is much longer and does not provide efficient stance phase and swing phase.

B. Endoskeletal: These are light weight and much rom is available when compared with exoskeletal. Cosmetically much accepted. The prostheis has adequate provision foe adjustments to achieve good dynamic alignment. It needs much less time for fabrication.

#### *8.4.4 Ankle and foot unit*

An ideal prosthetic foot should perform plantar flexion, dorsiflexion, inversion and eversion. It should stimulate muscle activity and shock absorber. It should provide a stable surface during stance phase.

Types of foot

A. Solid ankle cushion heel (SACH): It is the most common type. It has no articulation presents with solid heel made upof wood or metal , a cushion heel with rubber heel edge which gets compressed during heel strike. It has advantages of less maintenance, durable and light weight.

B. Madras foot: This is modified version of sach. It has space between heel and ground filled with sponge rubber, toes are shaped like normal and rubber sole is provided for bare foot walking.

C. Jaipur foot: It was developed by prof, pk sethi and team at sms medical college, Jaipur. It is modified version of sach in order to make it cheaper and cosmetic. But it has disadvantage it can be used only with shoes because the shapes of toes are not discernible. Advantages: It is cheaper, cosmetically well accepted, waterproof.

## 8.5 Application of prosthesis

### *8.5.1 Donning of prostheis*

1. Turn the sock inside out

2. Place the end of the sock against residual limb and roll on the sock with no air and wrinkles formed.

3. Adequate number of socks are needed to fit the socket appropriately

4. Place the residual limb inside the socket and try to ensure that the foot is correctly placed.

5. Push the residual limb into the socket .there should be mild resistance while applying prostheis. If there is no resistance then it indicates that less number of socks being used. So ensure adewuate number of socks

6. Check the knee cap in relation with the socket.

7. Buckle the suspension. Keep checking throughout the day for any discomfort or pain.

### *8.5.2 Doffing the prosthesis*

1. Remove the one way valve at the end of the socet and pull the limb out of the socket.

2. Remove the socks and check for any skin irritation or damage [6].

# 9. Syme's amputation

Syme's amputation (SA) includes ankle disarticulation which is done at the level of the ankle joint in which there is removal of malleoli and the heel pad is protected. It is performed based on indications particularly in pediatric population. SA has the advantage of permitting weight bearing without prosthesis.

Indications:

- Foot trauma

- Diseased tissue/ non-usuable foot

- Infection

- Tumors

- Certain limb deformities which needs excision

### 9.1 Prosthetic considerations

Syme's level of amputation needs to encompass on several objectives for prosthetic management. It should pay back for the missing foot along with ankle motion which provides propulsive energy during ambulation. Limb length discrepancy (LLD) should be considered before preparing of prosthesis has it needs to suspend during the swing phase of the individual during gait.

Essential socket fit will maintain fat pad beneath the distal end of the tibia and fibula. SA has many functional advantages but when suggested with prosthesis it has various cosmetic limitations depending upon the shape and nature of the limb being treated.

In Biomechanical aspect, the prosthesis must provide comfortable transition, minimize shear and provide comfort for gait.

### 9.2 Types & parts

Currently four types of basically designed prostheses are used for SA.

*The Canadian design or posterior door design*, also used for Chopart's amputation is the commonly used prosthesis for individuals with large or bulbous residual limbs. Disadvantages of this prosthesis is heavier in weight when considered as a cosmetic option.

*Medial door design* (**Figure 6**) is a commonly used prostheis. It has great suspension due to intimate construction nature of the socket. It consists of an expandable door made up of an elastic sleeve which improves cosmesis and helps in donning and doffing process.

*An expandable inner liner which is enclosed within the rigid outer shell*. It has a hidden-panel expandable wall which is used for small distal ends.

*Preparatory prosthesis which consists of a removable foam liner* (**Figure 7**) that interfaces with the external socket. This allows or has the ability to modify accordingly further allowing for atrophy during maturation process by using the patellar tendon to assist by unloading the limb. It is lightweight and easily adjustable hence considered as the one with great cosmesis. Proximal region at the level of patella tendon or below can be trimmed as the amputee progresses with limb maturation.

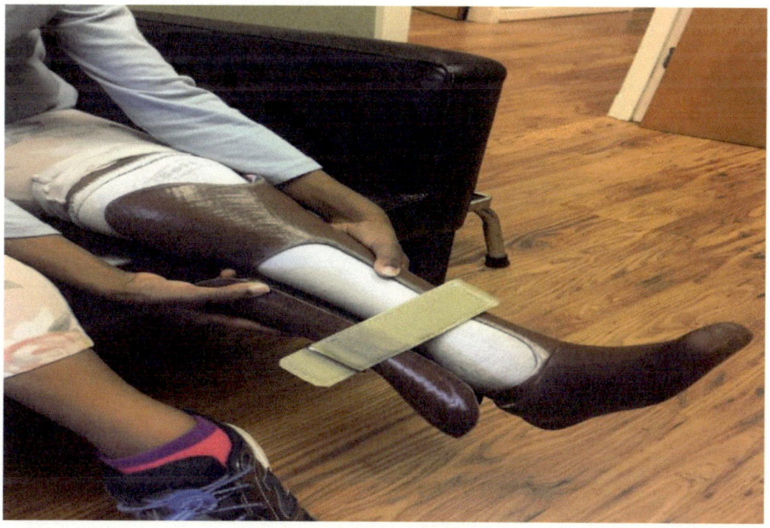

**Figure 6.**
*Medial door design.*

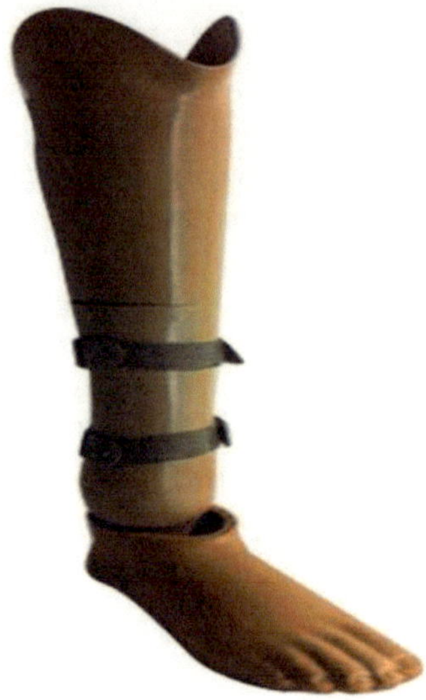

**Figure 7.**
*Rigid outer shell.*

A modified Jones compression dressing is used postoperatively to control edema and to help shape the stump [7].

## 10. Rehabilitation

The main aim of rehabilitation followed by a lower limb amputation is to restore daily activities by means of gait. In order to acquire full accomplishment the patient

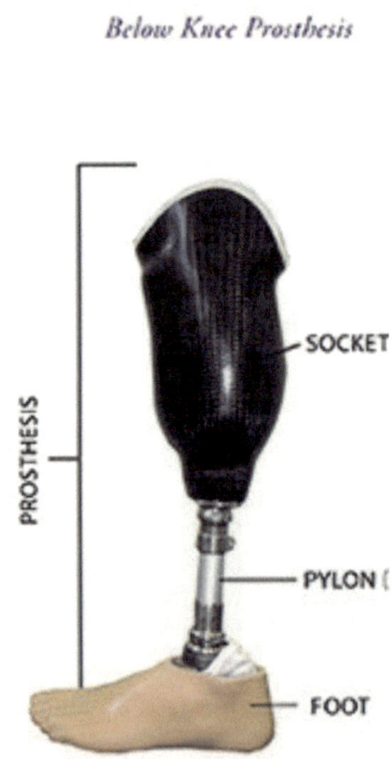


**Figure 8.**
*BK Socket.*

must be trained psychologically to obtain physical performances without any hindrance (**Figure 8**).

Donning- Initially the patient is demonstrated with fitting step. Initial fitting refers to the very first time the individual wears the prosthesis and stands, during which; patient should be stable enough to overcome disappointment about amputation and get adjusted to the prosthesis. Any discomfort should be immediately reported to the prosthetist. It is considered as the initial communication between prosthetist and the patient which will be followed by gait training.

Doffing- The patient is likely advised to sit down and remove the socket by slipping it off from the residual limb. After removal instruct the patient to check for any signs of ulcer or skin breakdown [8].

### 10.1 Prosthetic gait training

1. **Contents of training**: It takes several months so provide the patient with a detailed menu for the entire program from basic to advance. This will anticipate the patient about their progression and helps in self motivation. The menu can be classified into three sections:

   A. *Preparation for prosthetic gait training*

   - Maintain and improve range of motion
   - improve muscle strength
   - balance training along with single leg standing using parallel bars or a walker.

   B. *Basic training for prosthetic gait*

   - Balance and Gait using assistive devices (walker or crutch)
   - gait training within parallel bars.
   - Hygienic management of the prosthesis.

   C. *Advanced training for prosthetic gait*

   - Stairs - Outdoor gait (on rough road, slope)
   - Sports and recreation

2. **Residual limb changes**

   Explain about socket fitting and how it may change as the limb matures. As gait training progresses edema of the residual limb will be reduced, and it may fluctuate between morning and evening. Educating the patients about self management post discharge regarding adjustment of the fitting and maintaining hygiene.

3. **Adjustment of the lower limb prosthesis**

   Instruct patients about the alignment of the prosthesis which varies according to the weight loaded during gait. Educate them to adjust accordingly to avoid pain.

4. **Daily Life after the Gait Acquisition**

Provide the patient with a complete rehabilitation program.

*Precautions in daily life*

Even though there is a rehabilitation team supporting and encouraging the patient still it is difficult for the patient to overcome certain circumstances. Therefore, it is the patient's capability to withstand and progress further with continuous use of prosthesis by maintain body weight and residual limb related problems.

## 11. Discussion

All types of prosthesis are well explained with their application and advantages. Each prosthesis has its own uniqueness and the patient will be well rehabilitated with those prosthesis. Not all the patients are permitted into rehabilitation stage. It depends on factors like age, built of the patient, involvement of the limb (bilateral or unilateral), Psychology of the patient, socio-economical status of the patient. A multi- specialist Rehabilitation team has to be set to rehabilitate the Amputee.

### 11.1 Biomechanical principles of prosthesis and gait in prosthetic leg

The gait cycle which consists of two stages will also be termed as walking cycle. Initial contact is the first step in the starting point and the end point in every gait cycle. A single gait cycle has two phases. The stance phase and the swing phase. The stance phase is the initial step in which the foot contact starts followed by other steps in the ground. The stance phases contribute about 60% of the gait cycle and the swing phase contributes about 40% of the gait cycle. The swing denotes the single leg support in which the foot is off the ground.

The pattern of gait in subjects with prosthesis will present an altered gait pattern. Here the foot contact on the ground and the weight distribution on the foot is the key factor to be noted. The foot contact will occur on the heel in such a way the walking cycle will be as natural as possible. In this situation the sole of the foot will contact the ground and the weight is transmitted to the foot. Thus, the selection of foot component and the knee joint must be proper. This is because this will have an influence on the subject's gait when he turns on to the next phase [9].

During swing phase, the knee function is so important so that the mobility on the knee joint performing both flexion and extension facilitating the foot transition from plantar flexion to dorsiflexion i.e toe elevation. This will prevent the subject from stumbling and subsequent fall.

The residual limb must be placed on the socket which provides rigid and stable attachment to the limb. This aids control over the subject's limb during walking. The prosthesis socket can be divided into 3 parts. The top region of the socket is known as seating face. The central part of the socket is the primary control area. The function of the central part is to ensure correct movement and restrain it in the PA direction during walking. The last part is the distal socket end. This part will transfer only 10% of the subject weight to avoid abnormal weight transfer and this will cause subsequent damage to the soft tissues. The socket must be able to transfer the load thereby it ensures good stability of the subject's gait with better control [10].

During standing, there will be a stretching of gluteus medius muscle. This will maintain the pelvis in a balanced position. For a subject with lower limb amputation this pelvis position is taken care by the prosthetic socket. In a transverse oval socket of transfemoral prosthesis, the pressure on the distal femur end increases and the body is excessively bending aside to reduce the pressure. It is a non-physiological load transfer, as the load is transferred through the tuberosity of the ischium which reduces the arm of the exerted force and the overturning moments are increased.

If there is any problem in procedure of construction and principles in aligning the prosthesis, there will be an abnormal deviation that may develop during gait. This gait deviations uses more energy expenditure during walking. Once this is practiced as a routine, may result in over use of certain muscle groups which also causes muscle imbalance.

In most cases, the improper construction of the transfemoral prosthesis and transtibial prosthesis includes

1. On circumduction, the foot swings outward which increases resistance to knee flexion with prosthesis. Here the prosthesis knee flexion has been limited for a reason. Thus, the subject has developed the avoidance mechanism.

2. The lateral flexion of the spine, the subject presents a leaning gait with the shoulder depressed towards the affected side. This is due to prosthetic foot is outset greater than 25mm, incorrect prosthesis length, insufficient adduction or amputee sensitivity.

3. Excessive heel raise, where the heel of the prosthetic foot comes up too far and too quickly. This is due to prosthetic knee flexion resistance is inadequate for the patient.

4. Drop off during the late stance, the subject presents excessive knee flexion. This is due to softness of the keel of the prosthetic foot. Also, the toe lever of the foot is too short of the heel height of the shoe is too high.

5. Foot slap, this occurs along with rapid and abnormal plantar flexion movement immediately after heel contact. This is due to insufficient resistance to plantar flexion on the prosthetic foot.

Thus, if there is an improper prosthetic fitting, there will be pain and altered muscle activity during execution of the normal daily activities. This pain may cause lateral asymmetry of the body which is due to incorrect length of the prosthesis or incorrect selection of the prosthetic component. This wrong construction can lead to abnormal force transmission, overloading the various muscles involved and also damage to the soft tissues which may affect the integration of the stump function.

## 12. Conclusion

Thus, this chapter gives us knowledge about the types, application, advantages, and disadvantages of Prosthesis for lower limb amputation. The biomechanics and Gait through Prosthetic leg is also explained for the readers. There are few limitations in this chapter. The content on latest Prosthetic application through Robotics, Myoelectrical prosthesis are not included in this chapter. Further research has to be done on these contents to include in further revision of the chapter. Thus the chapter is fully concentrated on prosthesis for lower limb amputation with its types and application.

**Author details**

P. Senthil Selvam*, M. Sandhiya, K. Chandrasekaran, D. Hepzibah Rubella and S. Karthikeyan
Vels Institute of Science, Technology and Advanced Studies (VISTAS), Chennai, India

*Address all correspondence to: hodphysiotherapy@velsuniv.ac.in

## References

[1] "Text book of Orthopaedics" – JAYPEE BROTHERS, 3rd ed – by JOHN EBNEZAR.

[2] "Therapy for Amputees" – CHURCHILL LIVINGSTONE, 3rd ed by BARBARA ENGSTROM.

[3] "Amputation and Prosthetics – A case study report" – JAYPEE BROTHERS, 2nd ed by BELLA J.MAY.

[4] Ernesto Guerra, Jorge H. Nunez, Judith Sanchez-Raya, Almudena Crespo Fresno 2018.Prosthetic limb options for below and above knee amputations: making the correct choice for the right patient.current trauma reports 4(4):1-9.

[5] Christopher S.Crowel, Kte A, Impastatol, Alex C. Donaghy, Caryn Earl, Janna L.Friendly, Kari A. Keys. Prosthetic and orthotic options for lower extremity amputation and reconstruction. plast Aesthet Res 2019; 6:4 .

[6] Joan E.Edelstein MA, PT, FISPO, CPed -Lower- Limb Prosthetics and Orthotics- Clinical Concepts, Slack incorporated, e book

[7] Orthotics & Prosthetics in Rehabilitation, 4th Edition - Kevin Chui

[8] Article : FOOTCAREMD from American Orthopaedic Foot & Society.

[9] "orthotics and prosthetics rehabilitation" Michelle M. Lusardi, Milagros Jorge 3rdd edition

[10] Bernard O'Keeffe and Shraddha rout et al "Prosthetic rehabilitation in the lower limb" Indian journal of plastic surgery

Chapter 3

# Audio-Vestibular Neurosensory Prosthetics: Origins, Expanding Indications and Future Directions

*Ashish Castellino and Mohan Kameswaran*


## Abstract

Approximately one-third of persons over 65 years are affected by disabling hearing loss. It is estimated that the number of people with disabling hearing loss will grow to 630 million by 2030 and maybe over 900 million by 2050. Deafness has significant consequences on many aspects of an individual's life, including their socioeconomic status, mental and physical well-being, educational and employment opportunities. When congenital or early in the developmental years, deafness results in a delay or loss of language acquisition. Deafness can result from damage or disease anywhere along the auditory pathway. Hearing prosthetic devices help restore hearing and the use of these devices depends on the degree and type of hearing loss. This chapter will give a brief account of the currently available prosthetic hearing solutions.


**Keywords:** auditory brainstem implant, auditory midbrain implant, bone conduction implant, cochlear implant, hearing aid, middle ear implant

## 1. Introduction: the neurosensory problem

The global burden of disabling hearing impairment is estimated at 466 million people (6.1% of the world's population) where 432 million (93%) of these are adults (242 million males, 190 million females) and 34 million (7%) children. It is estimated that the number of people with deafness will grow to 630 million by 2030 and maybe over 900 million by 2050 [1].

Hearing impairment has a significant bearing on many aspects of an individual's life, including their socioeconomic status, mental well-being, education and employment opportunities. Older people with moderate or more severe hearing loss were more likely to feel depressed and suffer with poor mental health [2]. The deaf child cannot listen to her or his mother and focus on an activity simultaneously since both inputs must be processed visually. In addition, the deaf child is unaware of sounds of the outside environment, and thus, is centered on self and own activities. This has consequences on the child's development of language, social skills and cognition [3].

Hearing impairment results from damage or disease anywhere along the auditory pathway. Surgical restoration of hearing involves procedures that range from ossicular reconstruction to implantation of devices which serve to assist the functioning of the auditory pathway. The prosthetic devices currently being used for restoration of hearing are classified based on their mode of action in **Figure 1**.

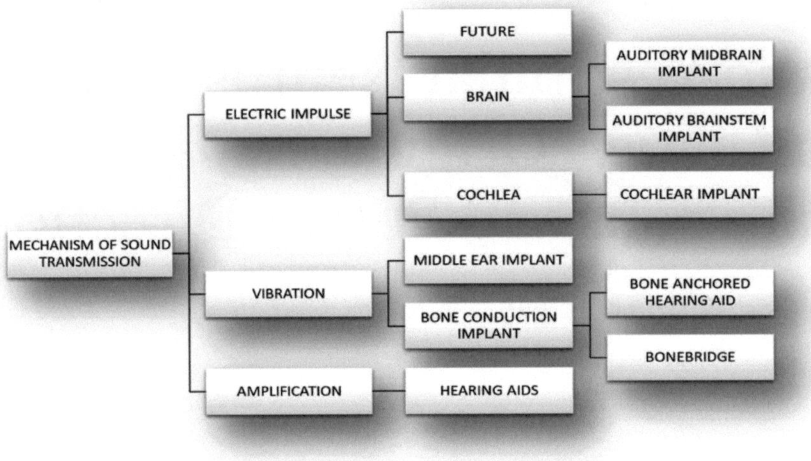


**Figure 1.**
*Classification of hearing prosthetic devices.*

## 2. The auditory prosthetic solutions

The first prosthetic used for the management of deafness on record in human history was the *Ear Trumpet or Horn*. These were funnel shaped devices which collected sound waves and led them into the ear, thus strengthening the impact of sound energy on the ear drum and improving hearing. The use of these devices date back to the 17th century with the earliest description given by the French Jesuit priest and mathematician Jean Leurechon in his work "*Recreations Mathematiques*" (1634). Commercial production of these devices began much later in the 1800s and many notable personalities of that era including pianist Ludwig van Beethoven are known to have used them.

### 2.1 Candidacy assessment

Hearing impaired individuals usually seek help only when they have reached a stage that they can no longer ignore their hearing loss. Often, it is not the individual themselves, but the family member/caretaker who notes that the concerned individual is struggling with their hearing impairment. In either situation, the pre-audiometric assessment which involves collection of relevant medical history and clinical examination of the hearing-impaired person is an important first step of the auditory rehabilitation process. It is important to identify patients in whom medical or non-prosthetic surgical management of their hearing loss should be attempted prior to dispensing of the hearing device. After the clinical assessment, the candidacy process involves a complete audiological evaluation using the following tests.

**Pure Tone Audiometry (PTA)** – This is a subjective test involving hearing threshold evaluation in both air conduction and bone conduction.

**Speech Audiometry** – This test provides information concerning hearing for speech, the type and degree of hearing impairment, and to check the reliability of the pure tone thresholds.

**Brainstem Evoked Response Audiometry (BERA)** – This test is an objective and non-invasive method of hearing assessment which detects electrical activity along the auditory pathway (from inner ear to inferior colliculus) in response to sound impulse.

**Oto-Acoustic Emissions (OAE)** – This involves recording of a low-level sound emitted by the cochlea either spontaneously or evoked by an auditory stimulus thus indicating integrity of the outer hair cells of the cochlea.

**Cortical Auditory Evoked Potentials (CAEP)** – This test is an objective and non-invasive assessment of electrical activity from the level of the inferior colliculus to the primary auditory cortex in response to sound stimulus.

**Aided Audiometry** – This test is similar to PTA but involving the estimation of hearing thresholds during the use of a hearing prosthesis.

## 2.2 The hearing aid (HA)

### *2.2.1 History*

The simplest and most widely used auditory prosthetic solution is the Hearing Aid. The first electronic hearing aids in the mid-19th century were large instruments that sat on a table. The subsequent invention of the transistor and miniature electron tubes made the hearing aid small enough to fit behind the ear. In the late 1960s the introduction of minicomputers opened the doors to real-time signal processing for people with hearing loss. Although not fast enough, these were computer-controlled analog systems which were used for amplification in hearing aid devices. In 1975, Daniel Graupe developed the first digital hearing aid in which high speed digital-array processors were used. This made it possible to process audio signals digitally in real time. Finally, in the early 1980s, the Central Institute of the Deaf (CID) developed the first practical wearable digital hearing aid which set precedent to the current type of aids in use [4].

### *2.2.2 Design*

The modern digital hearing aid is a marvel of sophisticated engineering and miniaturization. The microphone is the first component to receive the sound signal and it converts this energy into electricity. These microphones may be unidirectional, bidirectional or omnidirectional. A more sophisticated type of an omnidirectional microphone is an "adaptive directional microphone" which works together with the hearing aid's noise reduction technology to highlight speech sounds and important environmental sounds while suppressing background noise. These small signals generated by the microphone are sent to the amplifier which makes them more powerful. Compression amplifiers are used to amplify the signal while avoiding distortion and decreasing its dynamic range and can represent sound in either an analogue (mimicking acoustic waveforms) or digital (representing signals as a string of numbers) manner. The signal then goes through a filter which is used to change the relative amplitude of the high, mid and low frequency characteristics of a signal. Thus, the sound signal can be altered by the user or clinician to suit the type of hearing loss. Finally, the receiver converts this modified and amplified electrical signal back into sound with the help of electromagnetism which is similar to how headphones work. The hearing aid performs all these functions with the help of electrical power from a detachable battery. Based on where they are worn, hearing aids are classified as body (pocket aids), spectacle, behind-the-ear (BTE), in-the-ear (ITE), in-the-canal (ITC) and completely-in-canal (CIC). BTE are further classified based on location of the receiver as receiver-in-the-aid (RITA) where the receiver lies within the hearing aid case or receiver-in-the-ear (RITE) where the receiver lies within the ear canal.

### *2.2.3 Mode of action*

The primary mode of action of a hearing aid involves amplification of the input sound signal accompanied by frequency specific sound signal modulation to produce a tailormade output sound signal aimed at supporting the targeted hearing impairment. Hearing aid technology has seen rapid growth in the past 50 years and these advances can be broadly classified into three generations, all of which are currently commercially available. The first generation were simple analog hearing aids which were adjusted with screwdriver-controlled potentiometer trimmers according to the degree of hearing loss. An analog hearing aid consists of a microphone, preamplifier, a tone controller (or automatic gain controller - AGC), an amplifier and a receiver. In such devices, an acoustic signal is converted by the microphone into an electric signal which is amplified by a preamplifier and the frequency is shaped by the tone controller. This signal is then again amplified and converted into an acoustic output signal by the receiver. These were followed by second generation analog devices which could be digitally programmed by dedicated devices or computers. This involved coding of certain parameters of the analog components such as tone control and allowing these settings to be stored in a memory that can be modified or retrieved according to user preference. Digital hearing aids, which represent the third-generation, differ from the analog devices in that the amplified electronic signals are converted into digital signals which are processed by the Digital Signal Processor (DSP) before being converted back to analog electronic signals. Thus, these devices usually have an analog-to-digital converter, a digital signal processor and a digital-to-analog converter, of which the latter function is often embedded within the receiver in the newer devices. The entire system is built on a single integrated circuit that contains all the electronic parts i.e. transistors, capacitors and resistors [5].

### *2.2.4 Contralateral routing of signal (CROS)/binaural CROS (BiCROS)*

CROS are hearing aids worn bilaterally where the hearing aid on the affected side transmits the acoustic signal to the receiver in a hearing aid worn on the better hearing ear. In patients who have hearing loss in the better hearing ear, the hearing aid in the better ear can also be used to provide amplification to that ear in addition to the CROS input. This configuration is called BiCROS [6].

## **2.3 The bone conduction device (BCD)**

### *2.3.1 History*

In the 1st century, Pliny the Elder, a Roman scientist, was the first to remark about the potential of sound conduction through solid bodies. Several centuries later, Cardano demonstrated a method by which sound may be transmitted to the ear by means of the shaft of a spear held between one's teeth [7]. About a hundred years later, in the 1600s, it was Hieronymus Capivacci, an Italian physician, who realized the clinical significance of Cardano's observations. Using the same experiment he determined that if the patient heard the sound it indicated disease of the tympanic membrane, while if the patient could not hear the sound it indicated a lesion of the auditory nerve [8]. In 1757, Johann Jorissen, a German physician, published the first known dissertation dealing exclusively with hearing through teeth. But it was only in 1821, when the first primitive bone conduction device was developed by Jean-Marie Gaspard Itard, a French ear specialist who postulated that sound was conducted through the bones of the entire skull [9]. Using the concepts of the carbon microphone and the magnetic receiver (earphone) in 1920, Joseph Prenn of Boston, patented a mechanical bone-conductive ear [10]. However, it was Frederick Kranz of Illinois, who in 1925, patented the first real bone conduction vibrator which was handheld initially, and later attached to a headband and set the tone for bone conduction technology [11]. With the help of the Sonotone Company, Hugo Lieber developed a small wearable bone conduction receiver in 1933 [12]. Another idea was to fix the bone conduction device in eye glasses. From the 1960s to the 1990s, four different companies – Amplivox, Akumed, Otarion & Oticon made bone conduction eyeglasses which became the most widely used bone conduction hearing devices of that time. The idea to implant the vibrator into the mastoid bone originated in Sweden, after the pioneering work of the anatomist, Per-Ingvar Brånemark in bone rheology, where Anders Tjellström fitted the first 3 patients with the BAHA implant in 1977 [13].

#### *2.3.2 Design, mode of action & candidacy*

Bone conduction devices are prosthetic devices that aid hearing by converting sound energy into vibrational energy. The vibrations that are produced are transmitted to the skull bone, and then to the inner ear bypassing a hearing impairment in the external or middle ear, thus overcoming the air conduction defect. Below is a basic classification of bone conduction devices (BCD) based on their mode of action: *Direct-drive* (sound vibration is sent to bone directly in the presence of a skin defect), *Skin-drive* (where sound vibration is sent to bone via intact skin) & *In-the-mouth* (where sound vibration is sent to the teeth). BCDs can also be classified as *non-implantable* (conventional bone conduction devices) and *semi-implantable* devices (where some part of the device is implanted).

The **Conventional Skin-Drive Non-Implantable BCD**s usually consist of a processor attached to soft headbands (softbands), steel spring headbands or spectacles. Common drawbacks of these devices are that a high static skin pressure is required to transmit the vibrations to the cochlea, leaving the skin compressed for prolonged periods, which might lead to discomfort and skin problems. Also, skin attenuates the high-frequency sound signal and therefore sound that reaches the cochlea has a lower content of high frequencies. These devices are commonly used to confirm candidacy before formal implantation of a BCD. Alternatively, they are used when surgery is contraindicated or refused. Candidacy requirements for this type of BCD include a permanent conductive hearing loss secondary to microtia, atresia or syndromic; bilateral mixed hearing loss with bone conduction average of 35 dB or less and single sided deafness where bone conduction average is 15 dB or less in the better ear. There are no age restrictions. Below are some of the common conventional skin-drive non implantable BCDs available.

#### *2.3.3 The Cochlear BAHA SoundArc*

This is a conventional skin-drive non-implantable BCD that is designed to be worn behind the head with the BAHA sound processor attached to the connector disc just behind the ear.

#### *2.3.4 The Softband with BAHA processor attached*

This is a conventional skin-drive non-implantable BCD that consists of a bone conduction processor fitted on a soft headband and is indicated in the pediatric population with hearing loss as part of their pre-implant assessment till formal surgery.

*2.3.5 The Med-El ADHEAR*

This is a conventional skin-drive non-implantable BCD consisting of an adhesive adapter which is placed behind the pinna on the mastoid skin and a bone conduction processor which gets attached to that adapter.

The semi-implantable BCDs have several advantages over the conventional BCDs which include a lack of static skin compression and preservation of the high frequency signals. These BCDs are further classified as *direct-drive percutaneous* devices, *direct-drive active transcutaneous* devices (with an implanted transducer) and *skin-drive passive transcutaneous* devices (with an implanted magnet).

The **Semi-implantable Direct-drive Percutaneous BCD**s involve use of a biocompatible osseointegrated implant to which a percutaneous abutment is fixed. The sound processor is then clicked on to the abutment to activate hearing. The major benefit of these devices is an efficient percutaneous transmission of sound vibrations providing maximum amplification. Candidacy requirements for this type of BCD include a conductive hearing loss with an air bone gap of more than 30 dB; mixed hearing loss with a conductive component more than 30 dB and sensorineural component of up to 65 dB HL and single sided deafness where bone conduction average is 15 dB or less in the better ear. Suitable for ages 5 years and above.

*2.3.6 The Cochlear BAHA CONNECT*

The BAHA CONNECT system was the first commercially available bone conduction device. This direct-drive percutaneous system consists of a titanium implant which is osseointegrated into the skull, along with a sound processor which transmits these vibrations through a percutaneous abutment which connects the sound processor to the implant. The skin is left intact around the abutment using *'Dermalock'* technology. The Cochlear BAHA 5 sound processor features the *'BCDrive'* electromagnetic transducer. This transducer creates vibrations that are sent through to the cochlea via an abutment in the case of BAHA CONNECT, or an implanted and an external magnet in the case of BAHA ATTRACT (described later). This sound processor can also be used in the conventional way by connecting to either the Softband or the SoundArc. The BAHA 5 System consists of a range of sound processors including the BAHA 5 Sound Processor (for up to 45 dB SNHL), the BAHA 5 *Power* Sound Processor (for up to 55 dB SNHL) and the BAHA *SuperPower* Sound Processor (for up to 65 dB SNHL) which address different levels of hearing loss.

*2.3.7 The Oticon PONTO 4*

The Oticon PONTO 4 system is a direct-drive percutaneous device that consists of three parts – a 4 mm titanium implant that is surgically implanted into the skull, an abutment that is seamlessly placed percutaneously through the skin and a sound processor that clicks easily to the abutment and sits discreetly behind the ear. In addition to its remarkably small size, the PONTO 4 system also connects wirelessly to the internet using an IFTTT network.

The **Semi-implantable Skin-drive Passive Transcutaneous BCD**s have a major advantage in complete elimination of the soft tissue & skin complications of a percutaneous abutment but their disadvantages include the large artifact area on post-implant MRI scans and the possible dampening of high-frequency sound signals through the skin. Candidacy requirements for this type of BCD are similar to the direct drive percutaneous BCDs.

#### *2.3.8 The BAHA ATTRACT*

The BAHA ATTRACT system is a skin-drive passive transcutaneous device that transmits sound vibrations to the inner ear through a magnetic connection between the sound processor and the implant. The magnet which lies on the inside to the skin is attached to the underlying skull bone with a screw, and the BAHA sound processor is attached to a magnet plate on the skin via a soft pad to equalize the force distribution over the attachment surface. This BCD offers the benefit that there is no skin penetrating abutment, thus providing a good esthetic outcome with no need for daily care.

#### *2.3.9 Medtronic ALPHA 2 MPO*

The Medtronic ALPHA 2 MPO system is a skin-drive passive transcutaneous device that consists of a surgically implanted internal plate containing two airtight sealed magnets and the external digital sound processor coupled to the base plate containing twin magnets corresponding to the internal ones. In order to overcome the skin problems related to high static skin pressure, it uses a larger surface area so that the static force is widely distributed alleviating dermal compression [14].

In **Semi-implantable Direct-drive Active Transcutaneous BCDs**, the transducer is implanted in bone under intact skin. Hence, vibrations are transmitted directly from the transducer to the skull bone with the elimination of dermal impedance. These BCDs are labeled transcutaneous since it is an electromagnetic signal from the sound processor that is transmitted through the skin to the implanted transducer and not sound vibrations. Candidacy requirements for this type of BCD are similar to the direct drive percutaneous devices (except for age 12 years and above for Cochlear OSIA).

#### *2.3.10 The Med-El BONEBRIDGE*

The BONEBRIDGE is a direct-drive active transcutaneous system that consists of an external audio processor and an internal bone conduction implant. The internal component has a receiver coil, a magnet, a demodulator, and a cylindrically shaped bone-conduction floating mass transducer (BC-FMT) secured to the bone by two titanium screws. The power to drive the FMT is transmitted transcutaneously to the internal coil, processed by the demodulator and then relayed to the BC-FMT, which then transduces the signals into mechanical energy. Osseointegration of the titanium screws, however, is not thought to be crucial.

#### *2.3.11 The Cochlear OSIA*

The OSIA System is a direct-drive active transcutaneous system that uses a Piezo-Power transducer which sits within the OSI200 implant, and is positioned under the skin to send sound to the cochlea. The OSI200 implant is positioned on top of the bone and connected to the osseointegrated BI300 Implant which gives an important single-point transmission for sound to the skull. The system has a fitting range of 55 dB SNHL. The transducer functions on the principle of the "piezoelectric effect" which is the ability of certain materials to generate vibrations when provided with an electrical charge.

#### *2.3.12 In-the-mouth BCD: SoundBite*

This in-the-mouth BCD is neither direct-drive nor skin-drive. The vibrations are generated by a piezoelectric transducer and are transmitted through the teeth to the skull. SoundBite by Sonitus was mainly developed for single sided deafness patients. A microphone is placed behind the deaf ear and sound is sent wirelessly to an in-the-mouth transducer transmitting vibrations to the upper molar teeth. These vibrations are transmitted to the skull bone and received by the healthy cochlea. This device is currently only available for investigational use for the management of single sided deafness and is not available commercially [15].

## 2.4 The active middle ear implant (AMEI)

### *2.4.1 History*

Alvar Wilska, a Finnish physiologist, is credited with the first attempt at mechanical stimulation of the auditory system with the help of an electromagnetic driver. In 1935, he sprinkled iron filings on to the tympanic membrane of a patient lying on his side and placed a ear-phone over the man's ear that produced no sound, but an electromagnetic signal, and the patient reported hearing. Subsequently, in 1959, Rutschmann devised a method of fixing a tiny permanent magnet to the tympanic membrane at the umbo with water soluble glue. By introducing an alternating current he produced pure tones in the range of 2 kHz to 10 kHz [16]. In 1973, Goode and Glattke refined this work by introducing an electromagnetic coil on the postauricular skin to drive the magnet fixed on the umbo. Heide reported an important modification to these previous studies in 1988, by replacing the postauricular transducer with an in-the-canal electromagnetic induction coil located millimeters from a magnet fixed at the umbo [17]. Prior to this in 1986, Maniglia at Case Western Reserve University had already begun investigating one of the first contactless electromagnetic based middle ear implant systems. In that same year, Kartush and Tos, at the Michigan Ear Institute, collaborated with Smith & Nephew Richards, to create an electromagnetic-based partially implantable middle ear device that used an in-the-canal electromagnetic coil with a custom ear mold housing [18]. The use of piezoelectric crystals in middle ear implants became evident in 1984, when the RION device became the first commercially approved piezoelectric-based middle ear device to be implanted. Since this time, several additional middle ear implants have used this technology, including the Impex TICA and the Envoy Esteem. This was roughly a century after Piezoelectricity was first discovered by Jacques and Pierre Curie in 1880 after observing that certain solid substrates develop an electrical charge proportional to an applied mechanical stress. In 1996, Geoffrey Ball pioneered development of the VIBRANT SOUNDBRIDGE which became the first FDA approved Active Middle Ear Implant (AMEI) system for implantation in patients with SNHL, receiving approval in August 2000 [19].

### *2.4.2 Design, mode of action & candidacy*

These can be classified as *totally implantable* if all these parts are beneath the skin or *partially implantable* if only the receptor and transducer are implanted beneath the skin. Depending on the type of energy the transducer utilizes, MEI are classified as: *Piezoelectric* – when energy is transmitted to a piezoelectric crystal, which deforms it or changes its volume generating a vibratory signal; *Electromagnetic* – when energy is transmitted to a coil that generates an electromagnetic field that causes a magnet located close to the ossicular chain or the inner ear to vibrate and thus produce a vibratory signal; or; *Electromechanical* – which are similar to the electromagnetic implants but the coil and magnet are closely related to each other and the ossicular chain [20]. The main advantages of the AMEI over hearing aids is that they induce direct mechanical vibration of the ossicular chain or (and) the intracochlear fluids and thus generate greater functional gain, especially over the acute frequencies, with less distortion and feedback, increasing spoken-word discrimination. In terms of subjective results, patients report better intelligibility and quality of sound and a more natural perception of their own voice than obtained with hearing aids [21].

#### *2.4.3 The Med-El VIBRANT SOUNDBRIDGE*

The VIBRANT SOUNDBRIDGE (VSB) is currently the most widely implanted middle ear device worldwide. This AMEI consists of an externally worn processor that contains the microphone, electronic signal processor and battery and an implantable part called the Vibrating Ossicular Prosthesis (VORP). This VORP contains a magnet (that enables the external part to be coupled), a receiver unit, a demodulator (that filters the signal received), a conductor link for the electrical signal and a floating mass transducer (FMT). Sound signal received by the external audio processor is transmitted transcutaneously to the implanted device generating vibratory movements of the FMT and conduction of sound to the inner ear. The FMT coupled to the Incus is the original indication devised for patients with a healthy middle ear and moderate–severe sensorineural hearing loss in the higher frequencies with a discrimination >50% at conversational intensity who were not satisfied with their hearing aid or who had repeated external otitis. The VSB is the only AMEI approved for use in children since 2009. It is indicated in children with external auditory canal atresia and bilateral malformations of the ossicular chain who have sensorineural conductive or mixed hearing loss and meet the same audiological criteria as for adults.

#### *2.4.4 The Cochlear CARINA*

This is a totally implantable AMEI which consists of two parts, the electronic capsule that contains the microphone, the batteries, the digital processor and the connector, and the middle ear transducer that contains the receiver unit and the electromechanical transducer. All these parts are placed beneath the skin with no need for externally worn processors. This AMEI is indicated for adults with moderate to severe SNHL with a hearing threshold between 30 and 85dBHL especially in the higher frequencies.

#### *2.4.5 CODACS (direct acoustic Cochlear implant)*

The CODACS implant is a semi-implantable device that is still in a preliminary phase and is gradually being used in some European centers. This AMEI is indicated for patients with severe to profound mixed hearing loss due to otosclerosis either as a primary indication or after stapedial surgery has failed.

#### *2.4.6 The envoy ESTEEM implant*

The Envoy ESTEEM implant is a fully implantable device which is indicated in patients with moderate to severe and severe sensorineural hearing loss. The system uses two piezoelectric transducers (PZTs). Sound is received via a PZT sensor that picks up eardrum vibrations and transforms them into an electric signal. This signal is filtered, modified, amplified and transferred to a PZT driver which mechanically drives the stapes thus conducting sound to the inner ear. The sound processor also contains a power source, which is an implantable lithium iodide battery [22]. For candidacy, hearing thresholds should be stable and between 35 and 85dBHL for audiometric frequencies of 500-4000 Hz with a word recognition score of 40% or greater. It is currently indicated only in patients older than 18 years.

## 2.5 The Cochlear implant (CI)

### *2.5.1 History*

The history of the cochlear implant dates back to the first attempts at electrical hearing. The Italian scientist Alessandro Volta (1800) was the first to demonstrate that electric stimulation could directly evoke auditory sensations in humans when he invented the battery [23]. However electric stimulation of the auditory system was not subsequently reported for another 150 years until modern electronic technology appeared. SS Stevens and his colleagues conducted a series of studies to re-examine the electric stimulation of hearing using vacuum based tube oscillators and an amplifier, a copper wire serving as an electrode. They identified three mechanisms that were responsible - the first mechanism was called an "electromechanical effect" by Kiang & Moxon in 1972 in which electrical stimulation causes the hair cells in the cochlear to vibrate, resulting in a perceived tonal pitch at the signal frequency it was acoustically stimulated; the second mechanism occurs due to the tympanic membrane's conversion of the electric signal into an acoustic signal, resulting in a tonal pitch perception but at the doubled signal frequency; while, the third mechanism is due to direct electric activation of the auditory nerve. However, it was Andreev who first gave direct evidence of electric stimulation of the auditory nerve when hearing sensations were reported with electric stimulation in a deaf patient whose middle and inner ears were damaged [24]. The modern era of cochlear implants began when Djourno and Eyries successfully performed the electric stimulation of hearing in two deafened patients in 1957 [25]. Their success led to a frenzied increase in attempts to restore hearing to deaf people on the US west coast in the 1960 and 1970s. Although their methods were crude, these studies identified critical problems and limitations that needed to be considered and overcome for successful implementation of electric hearing. In 1984, the House 3 M single-electrode implant became the first Food and Drug Administration (FDA) approved device. This was followed by the Ineraid or Symbion device developed by the University of Utah, the Laura device developed by the University of Antwerp, and the Digisonix MX20 developed by the MXM laboratories in France. These devices were later phased out and are no longer commercially available [26]. At present, there are three major cochlear implant manufacturers including Med-El Corporation, Austria; Cochlear Corporation, Australia and Advanced Bionics, USA. In addition to its design, implantation criteria have evolved over the past decades. Niparko provides a detailed account of these evolving criteria in patient selection as well as the surgical, cost-utility, educational, pre and post-operative issues in cochlear implants [27]. Most notably, the audiological criteria for cochlear implantation has relaxed from bilateral total deafness (<110 dB HL) in the early 1980s to severe hearing loss (>70db HL) in the 1990s, and then to current suprathreshold speech based criteria (<50% open-set sentence recognition with properly fitted hearing aids).

### *2.5.2 Design, mode of action & candidacy*

The essential components of a cochlear implant are as follows – a microphone converts sound into an electrical signal for input to the speech processor. The processor transforms this electrical input into a set of stimuli for the implanted array of electrodes. These stimuli are sent to the electrodes via a transcutaneous link which involves encoding of the stimulus information for efficient radiofrequency transmission from an external transmitting coil to an internal (implanted) receiving coil. The signal received by the internal coil is decoded to specify the electrical stimuli for the electrode array. These electrical stimuli that stimulate the hair cells have signal characteristics which determine the sound quality of the perceived stimulus.

#### *2.5.3 Med-El SYNCHRONY CI*

The SYNCHRONY cochlear implant system consists of the SYNCHRONY 2 cochlear implant with the Sonnet 2 BTE or Rondo 2 sound processor. The implanted device has a removable magnet that may be temporarily taken out by a cochlear implant surgeon in the event that the MRI (up to 3.0 Tesla) is needed for the head. Med-El offers the largest selection of electrode options within the cochlear implant industry. Traditional electrode options include the standard array, medium array, compressed array and split electrodes array. The newest options include the FLEX 24, 28 and FLEX SOFT electrodes. The Sonnet 2 is a redesigned BTE sound processor for greater ease of use, better esthetics and improved reliability. It recognizes the ambient environment or scene and automatically adjusts settings to match it. The Rondo 2 is a unique sound processor option different from the Sonnet 2. It has innovative wireless charging, simple on/off button and automatically controls volume level for the recipient with up to 18 hours of battery life. The device is small and compact and sits on the head, just behind and above the ear and more comfortable to wear with glasses as compared to any BTE system.

#### *2.5.4 The advanced bionics NAIDA CI*

The HiRes Ultra 3D cochlear implant has a multi-magnet assembly which automatically provides alignment to the 3D MRI field, allowing adult and pediatric users to undergo 3.0 Tesla MRIs safely, without any preparation surgery or head bandaging. This unique magnet assembly is composed of four rotatable magnets encased in a revolving disc allowing alignment with the 3D MRI field. There is no need for head bandaging or possible surgical removal of the magnet. The electrode array options in Advanced Bionics include the HiFocus Mid-Scala electrode array – which is designed to lie in the center of the scala tympani in order to remain reasonable proximal to the modiolus (and cochlear neural elements) while not making physical contact with the delicate cochlear structures necessary to maintain residual hearing; and, the HiFocus Slim J electrode array – which is designed to be placed in the scala tympani toward the lateral cochlear wall away from the cochlear structures. The Naída CI Connect is a design-integrated solution which turns the Naída CI Q90 sound processor into a Bluetooth headset which allows for hands-free calling and direct audio streaming from any compatible device.

#### *2.5.5 Cochlear nucleus PROFILE PLUS CI*

Built on the same design of the predecessor Profile series, Profile Plus provides easier access to MRI at 1.5 Tesla and 3.0 Tesla without the need for compression or magnet removal. The Profile Plus is available with the following electrode types: Slim Modiolar (CI632), Slim Straight (CI622), Slim 20 (C624) & Contour Advance (CI612). The Contour advance electrode array has a perimodiolar design and a soft tip which is designed to reduce trauma to the delicate cochlear structures during insertion using the Advanced Off-Stylet (AOS) technique. The Straight array is recommended for patients with cochlear anomalies like the common cavity and in situations where there is fibrous tissue growth in the cochlea (bacterial meningitis).

The Cochlear NUCLEUS 7 Sound Processor is the smallest and lightest BTE hearing solution with built-in connectivity featuring direct streaming with a compatible Apple and Android device without attaching anything to the sound processor. The Kanso 2 Sound Processor is the smallest and lightest off-the ear solution available that has built-in technology offering direct streaming, control and connectivity with a compatible device.

#### *2.5.6 Candidacy*

Current clinical guidelines for implant candidacy represent a composite assessment of the individual's age (>12 months), hearing loss history, aided and unaided audition (comprehensive audiometric assessment), the socioeconomic and family support of the patient likely to influence the use of the device; and an awareness of potential benefits and constraints of current implantable technologies. These can be estimated via high resolution imaging complemented by thorough audiometric assessment and a multidisciplinary team-based preoperative counseling or intervention.

### 2.6 The auditory brainstem implant (ABI)

#### *2.6.1 History*

Hitselberger and House performed the first implantation of an ABI in 1979 [28]. It was a single spherical electrode implanted adjacent to the cochlear nucleus following removal of bilateral vestibular schwannomas of a patient with Neurofibromatosis Type 2 (NF2). In 1992, Cochlear Ltd. in conjunction with the Huntington Medical Research Institute developed the first multichannel electrode array devices which have, in most cases, provided patients with greater benefits than the earlier devices [29].

#### *2.6.2 Design, mode of action & candidacy*

Although in the earlier years the most frequent indication of an ABI was NF2, a genetic disorder with an autosomal dominant inheritance pattern in which the patient develops benign vestibular schwannomas on both eighth cranial nerves; in recent years, the indications for the ABI have expanded to include bilateral cochlear ossification, unilateral vestibular schwannoma with deafness in the contralateral ear that is not amenable to a cochlear implant, congenital cochlear nerve aplasia or hypoplasia, complete cochlear ossification, malformation of the inner ear, and bilateral traumatic avulsions or absence of the cochlear nerve [30]. The current ABI system utilizes 12 platinum disk electrodes aligned on a flexible silicone and polyester mesh backing for implantation into the lateral recess of the fourth ventricle on the cochlear nucleus of the brain. This bypasses a non-functioning auditory nerve and allows signals to be sent to the brain.

### 2.7 The auditory midbrain implant (AMI)

#### *2.7.1 History*

The first reported attempt at stimulation of the inferior colliculus (IC) of the midbrain for hearing restoration was in 1962 by Simmons and colleagues at Stanford University during a tumor removal operation [31]. The second attempt at stimulating the surface of the IC happened much later in 2005 and involved using an ABI array in a NF2 patient to assess if the limited performance with cochlear nucleus stimulation secondary to tumor related damage could be overcome by stimulation in a higher auditory center and they were successful in eliciting a response at much higher thresholds than what is used in cochlear nucleus stimulation [32]. In 2006, Thomas and Minoo Lenarz at the Hannover Medical University developed the first human prototype Auditory Midbrain Implant (AMI) array for penetrating stimulation across the tonotopic gradient of the central nucleus of the IC [33].

#### *2.7.2 Design, mode of action & candidacy*

The AMI is a type of central auditory prosthesis that targets midbrain regions beyond the cochlear nucleus, particularly the central nucleus of the Inferior Colliculus (ICC). There are several properties of the ICC that make it a logical choice for a prosthetic target including being a converging center for almost all ascending auditory projections, possessing tonotopic anatomical organization in addition to spatial organization for speech perception. The Cochlear Ltd. CI array was reduced in dimensions to create an AMI array that was small enough to insert into the ICC with the goal of stimulating its different layers. The AMI electrode array measures 6.4 mm long and a diameter of 0.4 mm and possesses 20 linearly spaced platinum ring electrodes. A distal Dacron mesh prevents over insertion of the electrode into the ICC during implantation and anchors the electrode array onto the surface of the inferior colliculus to minimize movement after positioning. The other components of the AMI system are similar to the Cochlear NUCLEUS CI system consisting of behind-the-ear microphone and processor that transmits the electromagnetic signals to the receiver stimulator implanted under the skin.

### **2.8 The vestibular implant**

#### *2.8.1 History*

Vestibular disorders are widely prevalent and can cause significant morbidity in the form of incapacitating symptoms, missed work days and even the inability to leave one's home. Advancements in the treatment of vestibular disorders are lacking and the surgical treatment of vestibular disorders has remained unchanged in the past two decades. Over the same duration, neural prosthesis have been developed that substitute one modality for another in order to restore a missing sense. Current research in vestibular neurostimulation has finally made possible the clinical reality of treating a wide range of vestibular disorders with electric stimulation.

#### *2.8.2 Design, mode of action & candidacy*

Vestibular implantation is useful in recurrent acute vertigo attacks (in which central compensation does not occur), for chronic bilateral hypofunction and for Meniere's disease, in which vertiginous attacks may be precipitated by an acute loss of vestibular tone. These are ideal candidates for a "pacemaker"-style vestibular implant that replaces the missing neural impulses during attacks. This implant bypasses the vestibular end organs to directly stimulate the vestibular nerve. The goal of vestibular implantation is to provide vestibular functionality and or reduce symptomatology by programmed stimulation of the vestibular nerve. This device consists of a modified Nucleus Freedom system. The receiver-stimulator has a modified trifurcating array of 9 electrodes. Each electrode is implanted 2.5 mm into the perilymphatic space of the semicircular canal adjacent to the ampullary nerve which is the site of stimulation.

## 3. Future directions

It would be expected that future devices will meet the existing basic requirements which include wearing comfort, cosmetic appeal, long battery life and customizable frequency-cum-level dependent gains for ideal hearing rehabilitation. There is extensive ongoing research in different aspects of hearing technology, some of which are described here. The micro-electrical–mechanical systems (MEMS) microphone allows for a further reduction in size as well as the possibility of multiple microphones on a single device. This will be very useful for noisy environments for selecting a target source while rejecting other competing sounds thus improving directionality of the hearing device [34]. Silicon microfabrication of microphones making them more sensitive and with lower thermal noise was inspired by the ears of the parasitoid fly, *Ormia ochracea* and is another unique approach [35]. As the size of the microphone progressively reduces, self-calibrating devices are likely to become more common in the future. Such systems can help in achieving target frequency-and-level dependent gains at the initial fitting and can greatly speed up the initial fitting process. Initiation of the hearing device could itself trigger a self-adjustment procedure to ensure the device overcomes daily variations [36]. DSPs have progressively shrunk in size and power requirement which together with improvements in battery technology will contribute to increased intervals between battery recharging. Developments in both battery chemistry and internal components such has anodes will likely result in longer battery life, faster recharging, smaller size and increased voltage that will enable increased dynamic range and DSP processor speed [36].

Bluetooth is one such technology that hearing device manufacturers are increasingly making available in their devices. This makes the hearing device compatible with any Bluetooth enabled technology across manufacturers allowing for hands-free usage of phone and other sound devices. Future hearing devices may contain sensors already existent in smart watches and other wearable devices which may collect information and present it via an auditory speech signal tailored to the wearer. There is evidence that auditory evoked electrical responses change depending on which sound source an individual is attending to [37]. This has been referred to as cognitively controlled hearing aids and research is ongoing in this field at present. The possibilities for improving the bone conduction device in the future are endless. A better housing design and improved transducer technology can improve conventional BCDs. This would be a significant advantage since they are non-invasive and a lower-cost alternative. Expanding surgical criteria to children below a certain age with smaller devices would likely offer them better hearing at a younger age and improved socio-linguistic development. Development of more patient optimized and powerful transducers will expand current indications for implantation.

A variety of approaches to regeneration or repair of auditory sensory and related structures are being investigated to restore hearing. Future hearing devices may be developed consisting of an acoustic hearing aid and a linked implanted component capable of eluting chemicals or signals for enhancement of this regenerative process. Drug delivery would be enabled through the implant, to preserve neurons or even promote the growth of neurites (toward the electrode array) from existing neurons or regeneration of neurons and associated structures [38, 39]. In 2002, the Free Electron Laser was used to conduct initial experiments on optical stimulation of a peripheral nerve [40]. This concept was later transferred to the cochlea and stimulation units have been further miniaturized and an implantable unit for stimulation in cat models is currently under work [41]. Necessary safety studies are underway that has led to the development of an optogenetic implant unit that is being used in clinical trials. The feasibility of supplementing the ABI array of surface electrodes with penetrating microstimulating electrodes has been demonstrated in animal studies and human trials involving using this combination is currently ongoing. The initial results of the first AMI patients have been encouraging in terms of the ability to implant the array into the auditory midbrain safely and to restore some hearing function. Future work in this area will needed to overcome the primary limitation of midbrain stimulation which is optimal placement of the electrode array. Research is also currently underway on creating a totally implantable vestibular implant in which all the components of the implant could be internalized. Advances in miniaturization, microelectromechanical systems (MEMS), nanotechnology, battery technology and circuit energy efficiency could help realize this goal. A vestibular brainstem implant could prove helpful for bilateral vestibular hypofunction and such a device could be potentially combined with an auditory brainstem device [29].

Thus, there are new development efforts in this field that will either significantly improve prosthetic performance or change the face of auditory prosthesis altogether. There is also the possibility that auditory prostheses will be integrated with other peripheral and central prostheses (eg. vestibular and deep brain implants) to treat not just one symptom but to address its whole spectrum. Finally, the progress in neuroscience, particularly in non-invasive brain monitoring will allow a full account of individual variability in both the optimization & the performance of prosthetic hearing devices.

## Author details

Ashish Castellino* and Mohan Kameswaran
Madras ENT Research Foundation (P) Ltd, Chennai, India

*Address all correspondence to: drashc@gmail.com

## References

[1] Davis AC, Hoffman HJ. Hearing loss: Rising prevalence and impact. *Bull World Health Organ*. Published online 2019. doi:10.2471/BLT.19.224683

[2] MI W, WJ S, SJ S, J K, GA K. Comparative impact of hearing and vision impairment on subsequent functioning. *J Am Geriatr Soc*. Published online 2001.

[3] URBAN E. Childhood Deafness: Compensatory deintegration of the self. *J Anal Psychol*. Published online 1989. doi:10.1111/j.1465-5922.1989.00143.x

[4] Levitt H. Digital hearing aids: Wheelbarrows to ear inserts. *ASHA Lead*. Published online 2007. doi:10.1044/leader.ftr4.12172007.28

[5] Holube I VTM. *Textbook of Hearing Aid Amplification*. 2nd ed. (Sandlin R E, ed.). Singular; 2000.

[6] Snapp H. Nonsurgical Management of Single-Sided Deafness: Contralateral Routing of Signal. *J Neurol Surgery, Part B Skull Base*. Published online 2019. doi:10.1055/s-0039-1677687

[7] Parisiis F& R. *Cardano G: De Subtilitate Libri XXI.*; 1550.

[8] Johannis, Beyeri H. *Capivacci H: Opera Omnia Cura*. Francofurti, Paltheniena; 1603.

[9] JMG I. *Traité Des Des Maladies de l'oreille et de l'audition*.; 1821.

[10] Prenn J. *Mechanical Bone-Conductive Ear*. US Patent 1346721

[11] Frederick Kranz. *Vibration Instrument for Bone Audition*. US Patent 1540783

[12] Hugo Lieber. *Hearing- Aid Device*. US Patent 1940553

[13] Tjellstrom A, Lindstrom J, Hallen O, Albrektsson T, Brånemark PI. Osseointegrated titanium implants in the temporal bone. A clinical study on bone-anchored hearing aids. *Am J Otol*. Published online 1981.

[14] Bernardeschi D, Russo FY, Nguyen Y, et al. Audiological Results and Quality of Life of Sophono Alpha 2 Transcutaneous Bone-Anchored Implant Users in Single-Sided Deafness. *Audiol Neurotol*. Published online 2016. doi:10.1159/000445344

[15] Hkansson B. The future of bone conduction hearing devices. *Adv Otorhinolaryngol*. Published online 2011. doi:10.1159/000323715

[16] Rutschmann J. Magnetic Audition—Auditory Stimulation by Means, of Alternating Magnetic Fields Acting on a, Permanent Magnet Fixed to the Eardrum. *IRE Trans Med Electron*. Published online 1959. doi:10.1109/IRET-ME.1959.5007893

[17] Heide H, Tatge G ST. Development of a semi-implantable hearing device. In: Suzuki I; Hoke M, ed. *Middle Ear Implant: Implantable Hearing Aids*. Basel: Karger; 1988:32-43.

[18] Kartush JM, Tos M. Electromagnetic ossicular augmentation device. *Otolaryngol Clin North Am*. Published online 1995. doi:10.1016/s0030-6665(20)30574-0

[19] Ball GR. The Vibrant Soundbridge: Design and development. *Adv Otorhinolaryngol*. Published online 2010. doi:10.1159/000318516

[20] Beleites T, Neudert M, Bornitz M, Zahnert T. Sound transfer of active middle ear implants. Otolaryngol Clin North Am. 2014;47(6):859-891. doi:10.1016/j.otc.2014.08.001

[21] Tysome JR, Moorthy R, Lee A, Jiang D, Fitzgerald O'Connor A. Systematic review of middle ear implants: Do they improve hearing as much as conventional hearing aids? *Otol Neurotol*. Published online 2010. doi:10.1097/MAO.0b013e3181db716c

[22] Maurer J, Savvas E. The Esteem system: A totally implantable hearing device. *Adv Otorhinolaryngol*. Published online 2010. doi:10.1159/000318523

[23] Marchese-Ragona R, Pendolino AL, Mudry A, Martini A. The Father of the Electrical Stimulation of the Ear. *Otol Neurotol*. Published online 2019. doi:10.1097/MAO.0000000000002153

[24] Andreev AM, Gersuni GV VA. On the electrical excitability of the human ear: on the effect of alternating currents on the affected auditory apparatus. *J Physiol USSR*. 1935;(18):250-265.

[25] Eisen MD. Djourno, eyries, and the first implanted electrical neural stimulator to restore hearing. *Otol Neurotol*. Published online 2003. doi:10.1097/00129492-200305000-00025

[26] Zeng FG, Shannon R V. Loudness-coding mechanisms inferred from electric stimulation of the human auditory system. *Science (80- )*. Published online 1994. doi:10.1126/science.8160013

[27] Francis HW, Niparko JK. Cochlear implantation update. *Pediatr Clin North Am*. Published online 2003. doi:10.1016/S0031-3955(03)00034-8

[28] Edgerton BJ, House WF, Hitselberger W. Hearing by cochlear nucleus stimulation in humans. *Ann Otol Rhinol Laryngol*. Published online 1982.

[29] Schwartz MS, Otto SR, Shannon R V., Hitselberger WE, Brackmann DE. Auditory Brainstem Implants. *Neurotherapeutics*. Published online 2008. doi:10.1016/j.nurt.2007.10.068

[30] Colletti V, Carner M, Miorelli V, Guida M, Colletti L, Fiorino F. Auditory brainstem implant (ABI): New frontiers in adults and children. *Otolaryngol - Head Neck Surg*. Published online 2005. doi:10.1016/j.otohns.2005.03.022

[31] Simmons FB, Mongeon CJ, Lewis WR, Huntington DA. Electrical Stimulation of the acoustical nerve and the inferior colliculus. *Arch Otolaryngol*. Published online 1964. doi:10.1001/archotol.79.6.559

[32] Colletti V, Shannon R, Carner M, et al. The first successful case of hearing produced by electrical stimulation of the human midbrain. *Otol Neurotol*. Published online 2007. doi:10.1097/01.mao.0000247808.47712.02

[33] Lenarz T, Lim HH, Reuter G, Patrick JF, Lenarz M. The auditory midbrain implant: A new auditory prosthesis for neural deafness-concept and device description. *Otol Neurotol*. Published online 2006. doi:10.1097/01.mao.0000232010.01116.e9

[34] Lewis BJ, Moss B. MEMS Microphones, the Future for Hearing Aids. Analog Dialogue. 2013;47(11):3-5.

[35] Miles RN, Hoy RR. The development of a biologically-inspired directional microphone for hearing aids. Audiol Neurotol. 2005;11(2):86-94. doi:10.1159/000090681

[36] Popelka GR, Moore BCJ. Future Directions for Hearing Aid Development. Published online 2016:323-333. doi:10.1007/978-3-319-33036-5_11

[37] Mesgarani N, Chang EF. Selective cortical representation of attended speaker in multi-talker speech

perception. *Nature*. Published online 2012. doi:10.1038/nature11020

[38] Clark GM. Cochlear implants: climbing new mountains The Graham Fraser Memorial Lecture 2001. *Cochlear Implants Int*. Published online 2001. doi:10.1179/cim.2001.2.2.75

[39] Qun LX, Pirvola U, Saarma M, Ylikoski I J. Neurotrophic factors in the auditory periphery. In: *Annals of the New York Academy of Sciences*. ; 1999. doi:10.1111/j.1749-6632.1999.tb08649.x

[40] Wells J, Kao C, Konrad P, et al. Biophysical mechanisms of transient optical stimulation of peripheral nerve. *Biophys J.* Published online 2007. doi:10.1529/biophysj.107.104786

[41] Cao Z, Xu Y, Tan X, Richter C-P, Suematsu N, Robinson AM. Electrical and optical co-stimulation in the deaf white cat. In: ; 2018. doi:10.1117/12.2291839

Chapter 4

# Design and Fabrication of Prosthetic and Orthotic Product by 3D Printing

*Harish Kumar Banga, Parveen Kalra, Rajendra M. Belokar and Rajesh Kumar*

## Abstract

In the clinical field, 3D Printing producing is a progressive innovation for various applications, specifically on account of its capacity to customize. From bioprinting to the making of clinical items, for example, inserts, prostheses, or orthoses, it is having a significant effect. Given that there are many energizing activities and organizations in every one of these territories today we will present to you a positioning of the best 3D printed orthoses. Dissimilar to prostheses that supplant a non-existent piece of the body, orthoses are clinical gadgets that are made to settle, soothe, immobilize, control, or right a piece of the body. Since every patient is unique, 3D printing is especially appropriate for these kinds of items and gadgets. Requiring an orthotic or prosthetic item likely methods a work concentrated, tedious, and chaotic procedure. For makers, creating great fitting orthotic and prosthetic gadgets is costly and requires profoundly gifted staff. Patients can anticipate that to a lesser degree a hold up should get their gadget, fewer fittings, and improved sturdiness. Developing a comfortable, properly fitting prosthesis is not just a science, it is also an art. 3D printing has the power to take today's bespoke, artisanal manufacturing process and transform it into a highly repeatable and consistent process, which ultimately results in more effective clinics and better patient outcomes.

**Keywords:** additive manufacturing, mass customization, product development, prosthetic and orthotic

## 1. Introduction

The design of medical products is a huge industry worldwide, of which, a major interest has always been the design of orthotics and prosthetics. Orthotics are devices, which provide support or stabilize an affected part of the body. They are used in cases of reduced musculoskeletal functionality. In most of these cases, the orthotics are used as the external aid or body support [1]. However, these supports can be used internally in the form of rods and braces. The most widely used orthotics includes splints, braces, slings, compression sleeves, and insoles. There are some simple orthotic products that we use in daily life such as glasses or spectacles, but these have been transformed from simple disability products to a fashion icon [2]. The timeline of Additive Manufacturing process is shown in **Figure 1**.

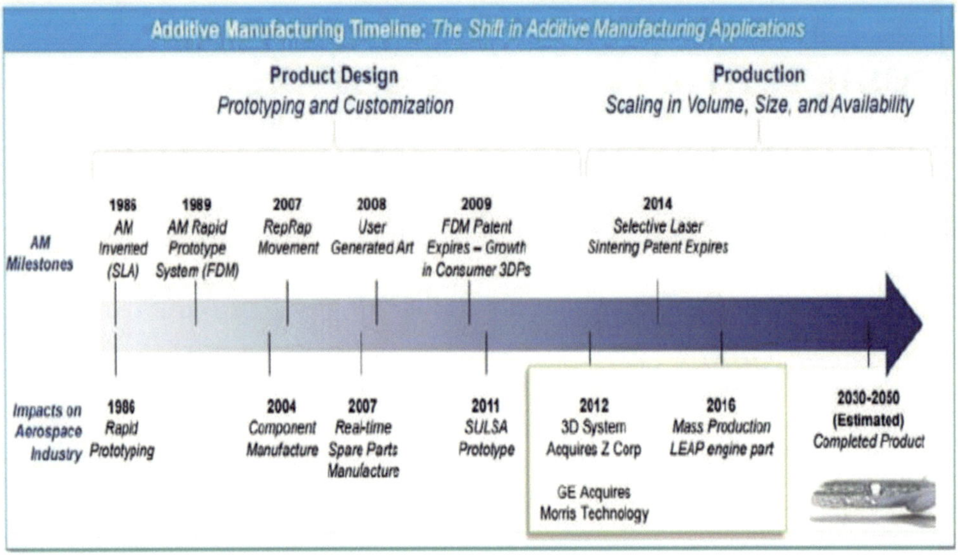


**Figure 1.**
*Additive manufacturing process timeline.*

Prosthetic devices replace or enhance the functionality of a body part [3]. They are used in cases of severe medical deformities or amputations. Other examples of prosthetic use include implants, artificial hearts and limbs. In previous studies, it is quite evident that the use of prosthetics not only aid the user by increasing mobility, but also helps in performing daily activities, thereby enhancing physical, social and emotional well-being [4]. The new science of "Prosthology" [5] deals with concept of the prosthetic part of the body being fully integrated as a new part of the body, as described by Gestalt's concept of totality [6].

Limb amputation has many disturbing and irritating impacts on patient psychology [7] often leading to stress and despair [8] Product design studies have suggested that the visual appearance of a product is one of the key elements affecting user choice and the product-user relationship. Visual esthetics also has the tendency to make products more acceptable and effectively usable in many cases [9]. However, this may differ across products and contexts. The overall appearance of a prosthetic limb is very important and may alter the level of the patient acceptance for the prosthesis [10]. However, in designing medical products, functionality is the designer's primary concern; with minimal attention given to product esthetics. This can affect user experience and satisfaction. Most of the available literature is focused on the technical and functional aspects of prosthetics, with only a few studies dedicated on esthetics, showing a lack of interest of designers and researchers in this area [11]. In the case of hand prosthesis, a previous study [12] also describes a prioritization of functional usage over esthetics. General steps of the 3D printing process as shown in **Figure 2**. While, another study by [13] suggests prosthetic appearance to be a factor that significantly influences the decision to wear or use a wearable prosthetics. The decision of whether or not to wear a prosthetic may be based on the user's life style and personal needs [14]. However, esthetics plays an important role in altering device adaptability. Additionally, if the prosthesis is purely functional but overly bulky, it can affect user acceptability and satisfaction. This can also have consequences which may affect the user's psychology state and social interactions skills [15]. In order to avoid such situations, it is important to focus on the esthetics of prosthetics.

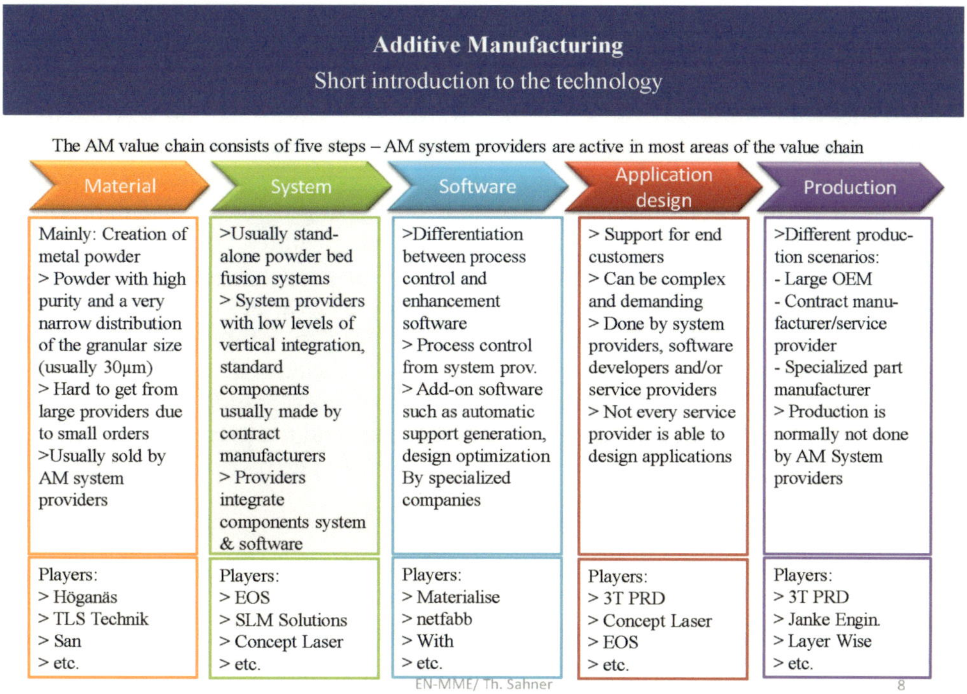


**Figure 2.**
*General steps of the 3D printing/additive manufacturing process.*

Several studies have shown that the acceptability of medical products can be improved significantly by addressing their esthetics [16]. However, a very limited number of studies have been conducted in the area of medical product design esthetics. The majority of these studies have mainly focused on improving the esthetics of upper and lower limb prosthetics [17]. There is still a wide range of possible medical products, whose designs can be optimized by improving their visual appearance and esthetic properties. In this paper, the authors explore the field of medical product esthetics. Some valuable suggestions and recommendations for medical product designers with the aim of improving user experience and satisfaction have also been discussed.

The joining of PC helped plan and assembling (CAD/CAM) has been around for fifty years. The innovation, which was initially evolved during the 1950s for use in the U.S. military, immediately spread to use by the car business. As the innovation filled in modernity, so did its applications. Today, CAD/CAM innovation is being utilized to produce everything from fine china and fly drive frameworks to-you got it-orthotic and prosthetic gadgets. Patients are as of now profiting by carefully planned and made cranial protective caps, AFOs, and numerous other orthotic applications, all or the majority of which have been made conceivable by the laser scanner, which has changed the manner in which shapes are caught and empowered massive advancement in the manners O&P professionals can think about their patients.

### 1.1 CAD/CAM technology in prosthetics and orthotics

The prosthetic and orthotic field has gone through huge changes with respect to innovative advances. PC supported plan (CAD) and PC helped fabricating (CAM), be that as it may, has increased just a moderate degree of acknowledgment in this field. Early programming programs were restricted in their capacity to exhibit to prosthetists that CAD-CAM was a successful device. As programming, equipment, and PC education increment, more specialists look to CAD-CAM to improve the effectiveness of their practices. New programming and equipment improvement ought to be embraced to advance acknowledgment of this innovation.

Computer Aided Design/Computer Aided Manufacturing is generally known as CAD/CAM, what's more, is an innovation that is used in prosthetics and orthotics. Foundation utilizes two strategies for CAD/CAM: one includes a fiberglass form which is then digitized into a PC for additional plan and assembling, while another strategy includes laser examining. The picture made is advanced and is three-dimensional. Foundation basically utilizes Biosculptor programming. Foundation utilizes CAD/CAM in prosthetics to catch the state of the leftover appendage, and in orthotics to catch the state of a patient's spine. With this exact picture, the specialist can change and address the shape electronically, and send the picture to our own profoundly qualified specialized staff for manufacture. The picture is then put away for future access.

For quite a long time, the manufacture of the prosthetic attachment has been a cautious and high quality workmanship endeavoring to make an agreeable, strong, and practical attachment for the remaining appendage. Through this attachment, the body's weight is moved to the rest of the prosthetic gadget and to the ground. It is the absolute most significant aspect of a prosthetic gadget, and the most individual and uniquely designed aspect of the prosthesis. As one would expect, there presently exists a huge scope of methods, styles, and ways of thinking on the best way to best make the attachment.

A careful form of the leftover appendage is certifiably not a decent attachment. The attachment must be precisely indented in territories that can all the more likely endure the exchange of powers, and the attachment must be soothed out away from the remaining appendage in zones that are less lenient towards power and weight. These uncommon regions of the attachment that require change are called locales.

Robotized innovation starts with getting an exact and reproducible advanced portrayal of the cut away appendage, and moving this computerized picture into a PC [11, 12]. Analysts actually banter the ideal method to "digitize" the remaining appendage, regardless of whether the appendage ought to be shaped with a cast or not, and whether the anatomic information ought to be acquired while weight bearing or not. Additionally, the level of exactness of the information keeps on being discussed. The primary effective frameworks utilized a hand-wrapped cast, which incorporated some conventional embellishment and alteration during the projecting cycle by the prosthetist. This prompts some variety in the beginning "computerized" map. In the event that a patient is casted multiple times, each cast and, in this way, each computerized guide will be marginally unique.

When the computerized portrayal of the remaining appendage is acquired, programming is utilized to include the alterations that change the advanced shape from a definite form of the cut off appendage, to the state of a working prosthetic attachment. This cycle is called amendment, and presents spaces on areas that can endure more weight, and help in districts that cannot endure weight also. Most programming bundles have layouts that will distinguish these locales and include these alterations likewise in any event, for various measured and formed appendages. There are in a real sense a great many varieties and speculations about the specific area and state of these areas, and on the best way to depict the inconspicuous subtleties of steady versus more sudden adjustment, and the area of the summit and the size of the change [13, 14]. Most programming bundles will permit an individual prosthetist to by and by refine the amendment cycle. Prosthetists can make their own layouts, so their top choice or best "corrections" can be imitated for different patients [15].

When the amendment cycle is finished, an altered model is cut, and an attachment manufactured over this model [14–16]. Once more, there exist an assortment of instruments for the manufacture of the attachment, and materials from which to create the attachment. While numerous prosthetists actually demand manufacturing every attachment inside their own office, the creation at this point do not should be done at the prosthetics office, and Central Fabrication locales exist to aid the various phases of the amendment and creation measure. When the attachment is conveyed, minor changes are frequently required, with the pounding or cushioning of little regions. The attachment then should be adjusted to ideally situate the leftover appendage according to the remainder of the prosthetic gadget, the weight bearing lines of power, and the ground.

The 1985 Special Issue of Prosthetics and Orthotics International- - CAD/CAM- - Computer Aided Design and Manufacturing catches and features huge numbers of the first ideas and thoughts from this time [11]. George Murdoch delineated the potential outcomes of making and fitting a few attachments surprisingly fast, and how this innovation will permit a professional and patient to investigate various ways of thinking of attachment plan or groundbreaking thoughts. He remarked on how this will build profitability of a prosthetist, and permit him to fit more patients in a given time. He additionally remarked on how this innovation will bring about improving the part of the handicapped in the creating scene: "there must be some reality in the fantasy that one prosthetist could quantify, manufacture, and fit many, numerous patients in about a solitary day."

Bo Klasson, likewise writing in 1985, gave a fantastic early on audit of CAD/CAM, and featured a significant number of the applications and points of interest of mechanized frameworks. Computerized frameworks can dodge duplication of work, improve considering three-dimensional math evading physical models, disentangle contribution of information for investigations and show of results, streamline documentation of the item, and store insight and data from past plans. He brought up that reproducibility will be a significant angle later on, and that the handcrafting fitting cycle is not reproducible. He likewise brought up the expected effect on instruction by changing over quiet information, which is picked up by training and experience yet is difficult to report, into verbalized information, which is clarified and dissected.

Klasson additionally talked about Gunnar Holmgren's high quality methodology and reasoning: that adjusting an attachment does not involve including or shaving endlessly a couple of millimeters anywhere, it is fairly a matter of changing the weight conveyances when making the cast. This discussion on projecting has proceeded. Klasson anticipated a Computer Aided Stump Measurement Technique, where the estimation procedure copies the embellishment cycle, effectively alters the shape, and reenacts the attachment before the estimation happens. This forecast has not yet become reality.

### 1.2 Current uses of cad/cam

So as to feature the wide scope of clinical employments of CAD/CAM in prosthetic practice, two offices were picked for in-house interviews. These two practices were picked in light of the fact that they speak to the closures of the range of CAD/CAM use. One is an enormous gathering practice that uses a full set-up of CAD/CAM gear to enhance in-house creation; the subsequent office is of an independent expert who limits overhead with an incredibly high utilization of focal manufacture.

The enormous private practice bunch has two workplaces, six suppliers, and two occupants. They possess and work a full in-house set-up of CAD/CAM gear, and accept the utilization of CAD to be their most effective model. The rule supplier initially bought a full in-house CAD framework in 1991. The next year, the gathering joined the utilization of another digitizer, beta test rendition of new programming, and another carver. This framework worked well until the finish of 1997, when the need to create spinal orthoses prompted the acquisition of an all-encompassing carver, digitizer, and redesign in programming. This update included changing over from a Macintosh framework to a PC framework. Tragically, the new overhauled framework was not completely utilitarian until mid 1999 when this gathering exchanged to an even fresher four-hub carver and a more current variant of programming. During this time of somewhat more than one year, the gathering returned exclusively to conventional manufacture strategies.

The current framework has been completely utilitarian for more than two years, and is utilized for creation of 95 percent of the TLSOs, 70% of the transtibial prostheses, and 40% of the transfemoral prostheses. Halfway foot, Syme, knee disarticulation, hip disarticulation, and all furthest point prostheses are finished by customary hand strategies. Transtibial prostheses start with a digitized hand cast, and every specialist has his/her own arrangement of layouts that function admirably for him/her. While the various experts all cast with marginally extraordinary method, their own inward consistency makes every specialist effective with his/her own arrangement of formats. For transfemoral prostheses, the ischial control attachments and elastomeric suspension attachments are made off CAD, while quadrilateral attachments and genuine attractions suspension attachments are made by hand.

This gathering creates around 30 TLSOs every month, and practically all are made utilizing the CAD framework. Strangely, essentially all TLSOs start with basic estimations, by-the-numbers method. Seven average/sidelong caliper estimations, seven circumferential estimations, and six length estimations are taken. The tourist spots are the navel (midsection), xyphoid, areola line, sternal score, ASIS line, pubis, and trochanteric line. This by-the-numbers approach has brought about a 95-to 98-percent effective first fitting, which is equivalent to the rate accomplished with the additional tedious inclined and recumbent projecting, and digitizing strategies. The specific, anatomic digitized detail is essentially not required for effective fitting of TLSOs in this predominately grown-up and injury populace. This gathering is as of now increasing some involvement in the new scoliosis conventions that depend on straightforward estimations, yet as of now digitize a hand cast for all scoliosis TLSOs.

## 2. Customary design attitude of ortho-prosthesis and need of esthetics

Conventionally, medical personnel such as doctors, physiotherapists and prosthetists are typically involved in the ortho-prosthetics' design process in order to ensure functionality. In the case of prosthetics and orthotics, functionality is important for enhancing mobility and fundamental in performing activities of daily living. However, the esthetic value of the product is generally neglected or only considered after the users functional requirements have been met [18]. Functionality is often considered as the cutoff requirement in process of designing medical products unless the product have some clear marketing value based on fashion and styling only. As the industry shifts towards user-centered designs, user experience has gained considerable importance and mainstream designers are increasingly aware of the impact. Hence, medical product designers now need to focus on product esthetics as well as functionality.

Today, we live in a world where bodily perfection and beauty are given a high priority. People who use medical products such as prosthetics encounter challenges related to esthetics such as social validation and acceptance [19]. Often unacceptance based on image and esthetics can cause feelings of social exclusion. Limb amputees face extreme difficulty in accepting new prosthetic modifications to their body [20], which can often lead to depression. Prosthetic users tend to avoid public exposure and are more prone to social isolation due to feelings of awkwardness and being self-conscious. These behaviors can affect psychological wellbeing, self-esteem and the ability to interact in social situations [21].

Design esthetics play a significant role in changing user behavior and product preference. A designer from Reebok theorized the value of good design by stating that "good design can make you fall in love with the product" [22]. Manufacturing process including Conventional and Additive processes as shown in **Figure 3**. By improvising upon esthetic features, users can have an opportunity to actively or to passively express themselves in their own unique way. Styling can enhance the acceptability of prosthetic usage among amputees by having positive psychological impacts. This can have positive effects on self-esteem and confidence. Hence, it is tremendously important to consider esthetics when designing medical products.

## 2.1 Parameters of esthetics affecting user experience

Incorporating natural elements in esthetic improves the user experience and acceptance. Many designers have used natural and organic elements in the product design process such as those found previously in Art Nouveau [23]. Organic elements not only mimic abstract human forms but can also be used as a stylistic element when designing prosthetics. Due to the level of craftsmanship and material handling involved, natural forms were considered to be difficult to manufacture. However, with emerging technology and ease of use of techniques like 3D scanning, modeling and printing, it has become possible to design and customize esthetically

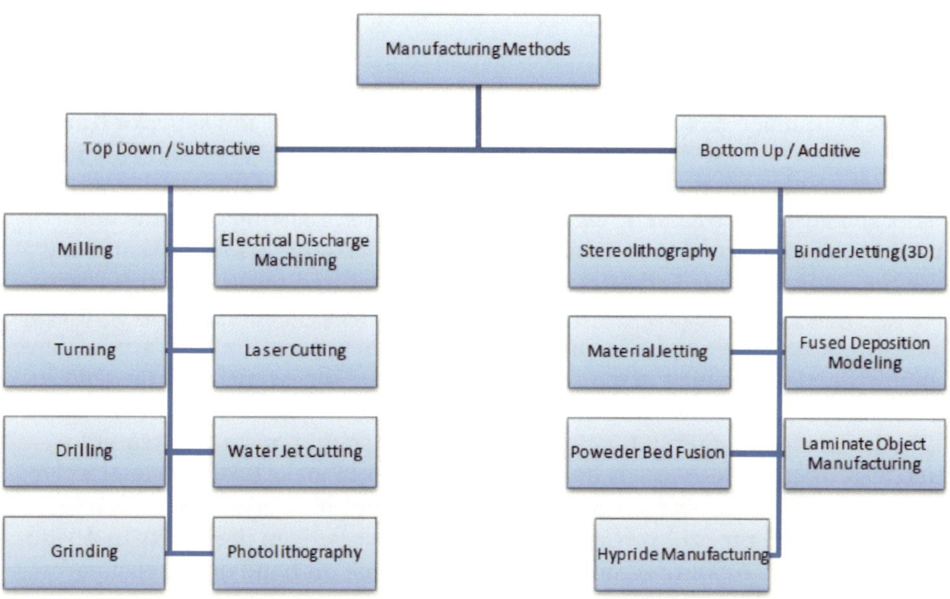


**Figure 3.**
*Manufacturing process including conventional and additive processes.*

pleasing medical orthotic and prosthetic devices based on personal preference. In the following sections, the authors attempt to explore the current esthetics issues of existing medical products and provide some possible suggestions and recommendations for improving these esthetic elements.

## 2.2 Shape and form

The shape and form of a medical device primarily defines its visual appearance. A study [22] attempted to investigate the factors affecting user satisfaction. They found that the most important factor suggested by the users was the shape of the device and how it matched the corresponding part of the body. For prosthetics, shape is an important element related to both functionality and esthetics. Another study [24] had similar findings. By exploring the relationship of Uncanny Valley and prosthetic devices. Uncanny valley is a hypothesized relationship between a prosthetic's human-likeliness and individual's emotional response to them. In the study, they selected 30 different designs with three different types of forms – artificial looking devices, devices with moderate human-likeness and devices with high human-likeness. Based on their results, the level of user attractiveness increased in proportion to the human-likeness of the device's form. This demonstrates the importance of designing devices with shapes that resemble or mimic real body parts. Conversely, other studies also suggest that this can generate negative moods instead of feelings of attraction [24]. Therefore, the impact of shape and form in the design process of ortho-prosthetics should be kept in considerate balance in order to promote user acceptability.

One of the key challenges in achieving an ideal product shape is the packaging and placement of functional elements (i.e., electro-mechanical components). For instance, some battery-powered medical devices, battery placement can be problematic if it is not considered during the design process. These elements can affect product esthetics and lead to user discomfort.

The workmanship and the development process also play a major roles in the form of the final product. With 3D scanning technology, it has now become possible to acquire accurate anthropometric data, which can be used to develop accurate digital human models [25]. It can also be used to develop highly customized medical products. With the continued improvement of 3D printing facilities, it becomes possible to produce such forms with a high level of precision and superior finishing.

Wearable art is one of the potential future trends in medical product manufacturing Wearables can be customized to fit a particular set of functional requirements and customary esthetic elements for every user. Existing orthotics and prosthetic devices could then be made to look like wearable art forms that blend with the users clothing. Esthetics and functions can fused together in this way to give psychological pleasure as well as the feeling of fashion and peculiar style sense. The esthetics of shape and form may differ based on gender. Previous studies have demonstrated differences in the choice of prosthetics that were based on gender perceptions.

In designing prosthetics for children, designers should make an attempt to stretch the boundaries of their imagination in order to make products interactive or in the form of wearable toys. Some research groups have also tried to develop Do It Yourself (DIY) types of prosthetics where the user is given the liberty to design their own device. A South African carpenter who lost his hand due to occupational hazards, sought a customized DIY prosthetic hand. He developed it using online resources and the help of a special effects artist. In addition to individual and laboratory-based applications, DIY prosthetics have also been developed as a manufacturing solution for amputees with the ubiquity and greater availability of more economical 3D printing facilities. The process of DIY ortho-prosthetic design and manufacturing can create new opportunities and facilitate in the design process of medical products.

### 2.3 Size and scale

The size of the product has a substantial impact on visual appearance. Size and material affect the weight of the device. If it is too large, it may cause discomfort and may be inconvenient for daily usage. Minimizing the size and visual prominence of prosthetics is important. Although reducing the size of a device may be more costly and technically challenging, it has a positive impact on patient's psychological well-being. Current braces have metallic parts, which are difficult to conceal under regular clothing. Smart textile materials can be used in place of metallic components to maintain product esthetics. However, if it is not possible to reduce size or to make a device more compact, then efforts should be allocated to make it unnoticeable and discrete in nature.

The size of a prosthetic should also conform to individual differences in body type to ensure that it maintains perfect symmetry with the contralateral part, side or limb. In order to develop products, which are generalizable and can be scaled according to a broader user base, it is important to understand individual variance in shape among the target audience. This can be accomplished by developing a database containing large anthropometric data samples based on country, location, ethnicity, age and gender of end users. Customization techniques like casting; last formation, which have been traditionally used, can be replaced by 3D scanning and modeling to achieve better results. In addition, modularity in ortho-prosthesis can be introduced at a grass root level to optimize device size and fitting. The concept of modular design can be implemented to achieve a "one size fits all" design methodology for mass production and may help to stabilize the user market.

### 2.4 Color

A lot of research has already been conducted on the relation between color, user perceptions and product selection. Although the range of color options for medical products is limited, still the color of the product contributes heavily in the product appearance.

In the case of orthotics, there is more flexibility to experiment with different colors compared to prosthetics. Depending on the application and user demands, products can be made transparent or incorporate color to stimulate concealing. The product design value for users changes when the product style or design parameters also change. For instance, traditional dental braces use metallic wiring to correct alignment issues. However, they are not esthetically pleasing and often make eating difficult for the user. Recently, several dental product manufacturers have started producing transparent dental braces without the slightest compromise on functionality. This example illustrates the influence of color preference in producing a positive user experience without sacrificing functionality.

With prosthetics, many users prefer the product to be similar to the tone of human skin. Due to the limited amount of color options for prosthetic devices, matching a user's skin color is challenging and may influence product acceptance. This could lead to a psychological unacceptance of the product as a part of their own body. Some users prefer their prosthetic devices to be more vibrant and colorful. Several new prosthetic limbs with printed artwork have been made available, which have been well received and successful among young users. Similarly researchers have tried introducing printed cartoon characters on orthotics designed for children which have been very effective. Body art's fashion trends such as tattooing are additional design possibilities whereby prosthetics can be perceived as more of a fashion statement rather than a reflection of personal limitation or disability. An intensive care must be taken to make the color of the device/product as natural and as iconic to meet the user's acceptability and psychological treat. The user should take certain cultural considerations into account when incorporating this type of device customization as it may not be appropriate for mass production. Interchangeable design skins may be a viable option in such circumstances. It is important to understand user needs and preferences when choosing the color of ortho-prosthetic devices.

## 2.5 Material and texture

Material selection is a key step in orthotic/prosthetic design. From the perspective of product design, material characteristics have a strong impact on the physical product. It is important to ensure the material selected has the necessary mechanical and physical properties required for the functional needs of the user. Concomitantly, careful consideration must be given when addressing more intangible characteristics like perceived values, personal associations and emotions. A study by, provides a detailed summary of key parameters to be considered by designers when selecting materials with a greater emphasis placed on the intangible characteristics of materials for improving the product design process. With advancements in material research and technology, it is possible, with new material options, to satisfy these intangible needs. Most medical prosthetic devices use metallic components to provide the necessary mechanical strength and polymers or plastics for the external encasing. Newly developed inert materials such as fiberglass, biopolymers and various metal alloys have been used to improve mechanical strength. The synchronization between user perception and product material should also be considered. Material texture preferences may be influenced by gender and various socio-cultural factors. Material, which mimics skin, may or may not be desirable depending upon the circumstances.

## 2.6 Adaptability to fashion and clothing

Just like physically fit human beings, people with special needs also have the desire to be perceived as attractive. An individual's appearance is highly affected by the style of clothing and fashion accessories being worn. However, the ability to use the prosthetic under fashionable clothing is an aspect often overlooked by medical practitioners when designing the device. Velcro straps can be used to affix bulky orthotic splints and braces which are often prominent, detract from personal esthetics and make it difficult to wear clothing over top. Due to bulkiness and prominent visibility of prosthetic devices, the range of clothing is limited Current design technologies have the ability to produce customized and sleek products which can be either hidden under clothes or can blend with an ensemble by matching the contour of an individual physique.

The majority of lower limb prosthetics are designed for wearing normal flat-soled footwear. This reduces the number of footwear options and may negatively alter the biomechanics of the prosthetics predisposing the user to postural imbalance and injury. Hence, there is a need for designing adjustable ankle prosthetics, which not only support body weight but can also adapt to different types of footwear. Following fashion and style trends are often important for the reasons of personal esthetic preferences. The aforementioned design considerations would help ortho-prosthetic users have greater autonomy and fewer limitations when it

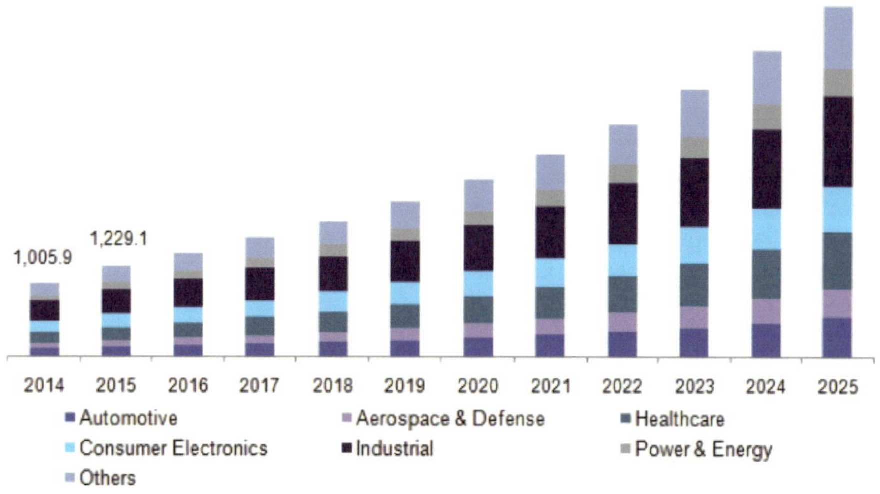


**Figure 4.**
*Industrial growth in worldwide by 3D printing process.*

comes to choice of clothing. This could have positive effects on social interactions psychological well-being and self-confidence.

### 2.7 Other factors

Factors like age, gender, cultural affiliations and personal attitude affect consumer esthetic tastes.Previous studies have shown that males prefer more masculine product patterns whereas females are more inclined towards products of beautiful and elegance. Regulatory and legal factors also affect material selection as products often needs to comply with standards approved by the Food and Drug Association (FDA). Industrial Growth in worldwide by 3D printing process as shown in **Figure 4**. Other factors, which also affect the design process, include the cost of manufacturing and affordability of the target users. However, esthetics should not be compromised based on manufacturing costs or material selection. Although traditional manufacturing processes help in producing more economical medical prosthetics in mass scale, 3D printing has proven to be highly cost effective concerning the customization of products. 3D printing can also avoid f material waste incurred during the casting and manufacturing process. In 100 addition, 3D printing techniques can be used to facilitate a modular development of ortho-prosthetic devices for individual customization.

## 3. Design approach – modular design

Modular designs are based on the concept of separating products into multiple parts, segments or modules that can be individually modified and customized. Recently, a large number of research contributions have been made in this particular area. A study done in 2014 proposed a similar approach, which they termed "Non-finito" product design. The products are intentionally unfinished giving users the option to customize and complete them based on their own personal choices and creativity. This kind of approach can help in achieving mass customization and facilitate product design flexibility based on individual preferences. Allowing users to be actively involved during the design process can help to initiate a better product-user relationship, which would better address the user's needs. This can also make the potential problems encountered in the design phase more visible to the designers. However, this type of design approach is seldom adopted in the field of medical product design. Therefore, the team attempted to incorporate the concept of a modular design approach without compromising the primary function (i.e., locomotion and movement) of the prosthetic limb. As previously discussed in the introduction, for the construction of the orthosis two important points are necessary, firstly, the scanned arm, and secondly, the anthropometric measurements. The first step to make the model in 3D, is to open the file in which the image of the scanned arm is located as shown in **Figure 5**.

Once the file is opened, the sketch of the measurements is drawn. For the sketch, three drawings are drawn, corresponding to each small size (S) measurement, which are, the perimeter of the forearm (plane 1), the perimeter of the wrist (plane 2) and the hand's breadth (plane 3)as shown in **Figure 6**. This way, the orthosis construction will be easier, since, to start from correctly adjusted measurements, a stabilizing orthosis will be achieved.

The structure has been created by surfaces, where the tool "lofted surface" has been used, and the 3 edges corresponding to the measurements have been selected. Then, the previously created surface has been thickened and part of the structure has been cut to achieve the desired esthetics. Also, the whole piece has been rounded off for a better result. Finally, a sketch has been made on the top face, where holes of random size and position are created, thanks to which better ventilation and hygiene will be possible.

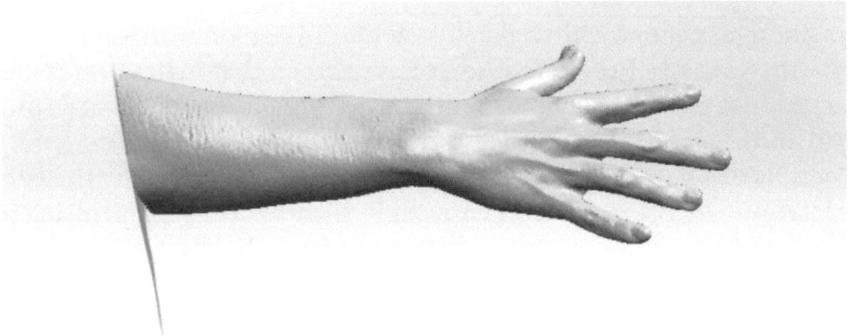

**Figure 5.**
*3D scanning of human hand.*

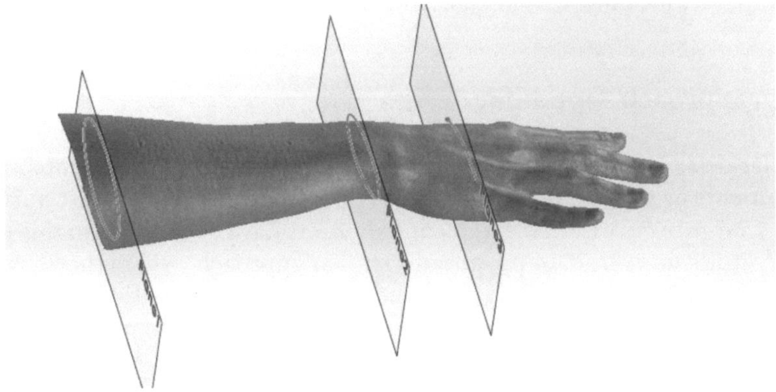

**Figure 6.**
*Sectioning of 3D scanning file.*

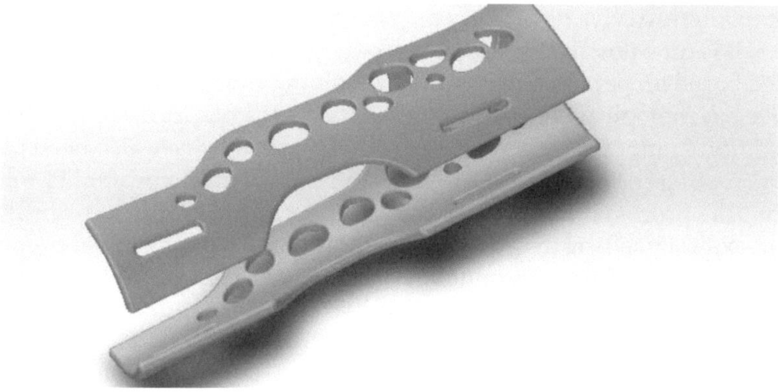

**Figure 7.**
*Final 3D printed prototype for hand support.*

Last but not least, the assembly is going to be made between the three components. The orthosis structure and the velcro bands are the parts of it, so a 3D model is going to be made. As final result it has been obtained a mass of 0,125 kg (125 g) as shown in **Figure 7**. A rather small value, so it can be said that the designed orthosis is a low weight orthosis, and that therefore it has been possible to satisfy the needs of a light and comfortable orthosis for the patient.

## 4. Result and discussion

Modular and DIY design approaches can help to address these issues by allowing the user to be more actively involved in the design process. With a modular design approach, it is possible to customize prosthetics based on the user's requirements. Users can also employ a DIY design approach by combining different prefabricated parts to manufacture their own product. This could facilitate the customization of such products on a mass scale. Additionally, designing ortho-prosthetic devices in the form of wearable art could revolutionize the field of medical product design and add an element of fashion to the customization process. Not only with this allow the user the option of incorporating their own sense of style or fashion into the development of their device but it can also create awareness for the inclusion of amputees across various social contexts. For ortho-prosthetic device users, better product esthetics are more than simply a means of flaunting or showing off, but means by which they can look and feel beautiful or be able to wear fashionable clothing like other people around them. Amputees have the same needs and desires as non-amputees. Meeting their needs is achievable when designers can give the opportunity to re-evaluate the ortho-prosthetic' design process with the objective of enhancing user acceptance in mind. It has been achieved a fairly simple esthetic, while innovative. This factor will make the product something attractive for sale, and therefore, it will stand out in the market. This esthetic has been chosen because the fact that it is a product for both genders as for all ages, so it is going to reach a greater number of people.

## 5. Conclusion

Allowing the end user to be more involved in the design process having user-oriented design (UOD) approach can improve upon conventional approaches to ortho-prosthetic device development. With the advent of modular design techniques, it is now possible to develop products, which are partially or entirely customized based on personal preference. Involving the user in the design process has positive psychological benefits and gives the user a platform for highlighting their creativity. Computer assisted design (CAD) systems have also been used to assist in creating the positive improving consistency and repeatability of this process, but the process remains slow and complex and it requires considerable input from experienced craftsmen. Furthermore, in these traditional processes the possibilities for innovation or product development are limited. With CAD systems it has been observed that orthoses rejection ratio has been reduced combined with time reduction up to 50% and cost saving up to 25% to 50%.

Maslow's hierarchy describes three different levels of user needs. These encompass basic, psychological and self-fulfillment needs. Traditional ortho-prosthetic devices address basic functional needs and allow the user to perform daily activities. Psychological well-being and self-fulfillment needs can also be met by addressing device esthetics. Ortho-prosthetic product design is a vast and constantly evolving field, which has undergone rapid growth. In past few decades, product designs for amputees have transformed from simple mechanical devices to highly sophisticated bionic devices. However, the esthetic features of these devices have received little consideration. Studies have shown that the absence of esthetics can have negative psychological and cognitive consequences for users. This study attempted to identify some of the key esthetic parameters, which influence the ortho-prosthetic design process. The authors have provided relevant suggestions and recommendations for addressing these issues with a modular design approach. A case study involving the design of a prosthetic limb socket was given to elucidate the benefits and implications of this user-centered approach. Developing a single product, which satisfies the needs of every individual user, is challenging. There are social, psychological, economic, cultural and personal preference factors, which influence user perception and experience.

## Declaration of conflicting interests

No potential conflicts of interest with respect to the research, authorship, and publication of this article as declared by Author(s).

## Funding

The author(s) received no financial support for the research, authorship, and publication of this article.

## Author details

Harish Kumar Banga[1*], Parveen Kalra[2], Rajendra M. Belokar[2] and Rajesh Kumar[3]

1 Department of Mechanical Engineering, Guru Nanak Dev Engineering College, Ludhiana, India

2 Department of Production and Industrial Engineering, Punjab Engineering College, Chandigarh, India

3 Department of Mechanical Engineering, UIET, Panjab University, Chandigarh, India

*Address all correspondence to: drhkbanga@gmail.com

## References


[1] Abboud, R. J.'Relevant Foot Biomechanics', *Current Orthopedics*, (2002), Vol. 6, pp165-179.

[2] Alexander, M. A., Xing, S. Y. & Bhagia, S. M Lower Limb Orthotics [Online]. *Webmd Llc.* (2011). Available: Http://Emedicine.Medscape.Com/Article/314838-Overview#Aw2aab6b5 [Accessed 22-09-2011].

[3] American Orthotic and Prosthetic Association Inc. Evidence Note( 2008) - 'The Use Of Ankle-Foot Orthoses In The Management of Stroke', Vol. 5 No. 12, pp.120-128.

[4] Banga, H.K., Kalra, P., Belokar, R.M. and Kumar, R. (2020), "Customized design and additive manufacturing of kids' ankle foot orthosis", Rapid Prototyping Journal, Vol. ahead-of-print No. ahead-of-print. https://doi.org/10.1108/RPJ-07-2019-0194

[5] Banga H.K., Kalra P., Belokar R.M., Kumar R. (2020) 'Effect of 3D-Printed Ankle Foot Orthosis During Walking of Foot Deformities Patients'. In: Kumar H., Jain P. (eds) *Recent Advances in Mechanical Engineering. Lecture Notes in Mechanical Engineering.* Springer, Singapore, pp 275-288

[6] Banga H.K., Kalra P., Belokar R.M., Kumar R. (2020) Role of Finite Element Analysis in Customized Design of Kid's Orthotic Product'. In: Singh S., Prakash C., Singh R. (eds) *Characterization, Testing, Measurement, and Metrology*, Pages 139-159 CRC Press Taylor & Francis, USA

[7] Banga H.K., Kalra P., Belokar R.M., Kumar R. (2020) Improvement of Human Gait in Foot Deformities Patients by 3D Printed Ankle–Foot Orthosis. In: Singh S., Prakash C., Singh R. (eds) *3D Printing in Biomedical Engineering. Materials Horizons: From Nature to Nanomaterials*. Springer, Singapor

[8] Banga H.K, Kalra Parveen, Belokar R.M, Kumar R, (2018)' Fabrication And Stress Analysis of Ankle Foot Orthosis With Additive Manufacturing', *Rapid prototyping journal, Emerald Publishing;* Vol. 24 No. 2, pp. 300-312.

[9] Boone DA, Burgess EM, Mathews D. (1997) The application of CAD/CAM in the developing world. In: Boenick U, Nader M, eds. International Symposium: CAD/CAM Systems in Pedorthics, *Prosthetics & Orthotics;* May 4-5, Nuremberg, Germany. p. 417-8.

[10] Boone DA, Urban ND, Smith DG, Burgess EM, Mathews DE, Coleman KL. (1998) Use of CAD/CAM for prosthetic services in the developing world. *Proceeding of the 9th World Congress of the International Society for Prosthetics and Orthotics*; June 30–July 3, Amsterdam, The Netherlands. p. 74-6.

[11] Boehler, W. & Marbs, A, (2002). '3D scanning instruments'. P*roceedings of the CIPA WG 6 International Workshop on Scanning for Cultural Heritage Recording*, Ziti, Thessaloniki. . Vol. 3 No. 12, pp 9-18.

[12] Branko Brackx, Michaël Van Damme, Arnout Matthys, Bram Vanderborght And Dirk Lefeber (2012) 'Passive Ankle-Foot Prosthesis Prototype With Extended Push-Off', *International Journal Of Advanced Robotic Systems.* Vol. 1 No. 10, pp 19-28.

[13] Bradford C. Bennett, Shawn D. Russell, and Mark F. Abel, (2012), 'The Effects Of Ankle Foot Orthoses On Energy Recovery And Work During Gait In Children With Cerebral Palsy', *Clin Biomech (Bristol, Avon).* March; Vol. 27 No.3 pp 287-291.

[14] Bregman, D. J. J., Rozumalski, A., Koops, D., De Groot, V., Schwartz, M. & Harlaar, J. (2009) 'A New Method For Evaluating Ankle-Foot Orthosis Characteristics', *Gait & Posture*, Vol. 30, No.6, pp144-149.

[15] Brehm, M.-A., Harlaar, J. & Schwartz, M. (2008) 'Effect Of Ankle-Foot Orthoses On Walking Efficiency And Gait In Children With Cerebral Palsy', *Journal Of Rehabilitation Medicine,* Vol. 4, No.9 pp 529-534.

[16] Bowker, P. (1993). 'Biomechanical basis of orthotic management', *Oxford England*; Vol. 2 No. 10, pp 19-28.

[17] Chen, C.-L., Yeung, K.-T., Wang, C.-H., Chu, H.-T. & Yeh, C.-Y. (1999) ' Anterior Ankle-Foot Orthosis Effects On Postural Stability In Hemiplegic Patients', *Archives of Physical Medicine And Rehabilitation*, Vol. 8 No.5,pp 1587-1592.

[18] Chu, T. M., Reddy, N. P. & Padovan, J. (1995), 'Three-Dimensional Finite Element Stress Analysis of the Polypropylene, Ankle-Foot Orthosis: Static Analysis', *Medical Engineering & Physics*, Vol. 17, No.5, pp372-379.

[19] Cook, D., Gervasi, V., Rizza, R., Kamara, S. & Xue-Cheng, L. 'Additive fabrication of custom pedorthoses for clubfoot correction', *Rapid Prototyping Journal*, (2010). Vol. 16, pp 189-193.

[20] Constantinos Mavroidis, Richard G Ranky, Mark L Sivak, Benjamin L Patritti, Joseph Dipisa, (2011), 'Patient Specific Ankle-Foot Orthoses Using Rapid Prototyping', *Journal Of Neuroengineering And Rehabilitation*. Vol.1, No.5, pp 252-259.

[21] Crabtree, C. A. & Higginson, J. S. (2009) 'Modeling Neuromuscular Effects of Ankle Foot Orthoses (AFO's) In Computer Simulations Of Gait', *Gait & Posture*, Vol. 29, pp 65-70.

[22] De Burgh, J. (2003) 'The Human Body - An Essential Guide To How The Body Works', *Rochester, U.K.,* Grange Books.

[23] Elisa S. Schrank, B. S. J. S., (2011). 'Dimensional accuracy of ankle-foot orthoses constructed by rapid customization and manufacturing framework', *Journal of Rehabilitation Research & Development*, Vol. 48, pp 31-42.

[24] Edelstein, J. E. & Bruckner, J. (2002) 'Orthotics: A Comprehensive Clinical Approach', *John Wiley & Sons New Jersey,* USA, Slack.

[25] Fan Gao, , William Carlton, Susan Kapp, (2009) 'Development Of A Motorized Device For Quantitative Investigation Of AFO's. Vol. 15, No.3, pp 112-119.

## Section 2

# Orthotics

Chapter 5

# Impact of Self-Selected Customized Orthotics on Lower Limbs Biomechanics

*Benjamin Dourthe, Judith Osterloh, Vinzenz Von Tscharner, Sandro Nigg and Benno M. Nigg*

## Abstract

Customized insoles are commonly prescribed to prevent or treat a variety of foot pathologies and to reduce foot and lower limb fatigue. Due to the patient-specific design and production of such orthotics, the concept of self-selected customized orthotics (SSCO) has recently been developed. The goal of this study was to assess the impact of SSCO technology on several physiological and biomechanical variables during uphill power walking. Thirty male participants underwent an uphill power walking intervention at constant speed in two insoles conditions (control and SSCO). The electromyographic (EMG) activity of their right gastrocnemii and vastii muscles was measured. Perceived fatigue was assessed every 5 minutes and the intervention stopped when the targeted fatigue level was reached. Baseline and post-intervention assessments were also performed. Sixty-three percent of the participants experienced an improvement in foot fatigue while wearing the SSCO. The foot arch seemed to collapse less when participants wore the SSCO, but statistical significance was not reached. The changes in mean EMG activity was not consistent between the 50% isometric contraction and the walking trial. In conclusion, while some interesting trends were observed when wearing SSCO, further investigations should be performed to try and reach statistical significance.

**Keywords:** orthopedics, custom orthotics, orthotics, lower limbs, insoles, walking, fatigue, neuromuscular, biomechanics

## 1. Introduction

Customized insoles have been shown to reduce pain [1], improve static balance [2] and redistribute pressure [3, 4]. As a result, they are commonly prescribed to prevent or treat a variety of foot pathologies [5]. For instance, wearing custom-made foot orthoses has been reported to reduce medial foot loading and/or improve the condition of people with patellofemoral pain [6]. Research has also shown that the use of custom-made laterally wedged insoles can reduce pain, enhance joint function and improve quality of life in older adults affected by medial knee osteoarthritis [7]. Customized insoles have also demonstrated the ability to prevent deformations and necrosis of the foot by decreasing forefoot pressure [8–12], hence reducing the risks of ulceration for patients with diabetes and neuropathy [13, 14]. Custom-made inserts can also be prescribed to reduce areas of peak pressure in individuals with high medial longitudinal arches, leading to a lower risk of developing pes cavus deformities [15].

Besides their ability to improve people's health, comfort and quality of life, customized insoles are also designed to reduce the sensation of foot and lower limbs fatigue. For example, see [16], investigated the effect of custom-made orthotics in healthy participants undergoing long periods of standing and walking at work. The results reported a significant reduction in foot fatigue reflected by 68% of the population experiencing less foot discomfort at the end of the day, and by 60% of the participants reporting more comfort at work when wearing customized orthotics. Another study by, see [15], studied the impact of customized insoles on a population of females with idiopathic pes cavus during gait. They reported that the integrated electromyography (EMG) activity of four leg muscles (i.e. tibialis anterior, gastrocnemius medialis, rectus femoris and biceps femoris) decreased after wearing the custom-made orthotics. Also, see [17], studied the impact of insoles with custom arch support during uphill and downhill walking for individuals with flatfoot conditions. Their findings showed that added arch support led to a significant decrease in peak oxygen uptake ($VO_2$), as well as a potential reduction in the activity of the rectus femoris. This indicates that wearing insoles with customized arch support could potentially improve motor control efficiency, and hence reduce fatigue in the lower extremities during gait.

In summary, multiple scientific evidence has demonstrated that custom-made insoles can positively impact people's health and quality of life. Yet, the patient specific design and production of such orthotics remains a potential limitation. Due to the known deformability of the foot [18–20], customized orthotics were originally molded based on a foot cast taken under different weight-bearing conditions [3]. With the constant advancements in 3D scanning and 3D printing technologies, the development of customized insoles is now being facilitated by the combined use of computer-aided design and computer-aided manufacturing (CAD-CAM). Nevertheless, the design and production of custom-made orthotics still require an in-depth examination with a specialist involving a variety of measurements, which can be time-consuming and potentially costly.

As a result, the concept of self-selected customized orthotics (SSCO) has recently been developed and introduced in stores and pharmacies. This concept is based on the use of an automated kiosk (Dr. Scholl's®, Bayer Healthcare, LLC, Whippany, NJ, USA) with embedded plantar pressure scan that can measure foot size, arch type and weight. Using the corresponding measures, the kiosk's recommendation engine can pre-select a specific insole design among a finite set of prefabricated orthotics with different arch and heel support characteristics. Such a system could represent an interesting opportunity to extend the accessibility of customized insole technology. However, conversely to traditional custom-made insoles, no investigation has yet measured the potential benefits of wearing SSCO. This study was designed to assess the impact of this new insole technology on several physiological and biomechanical variables during gait. More specifically, this study focuses on how SSCO can potentially reduce the perception of fatigue during uphill power walking.

## 2. Methods

### 2.1 Recruitment and testing conditions

This study was approved by the Conjoint Health Research Ethics Board of the University of Calgary (Ref: REB17-0875_MOD5). A total of 30 male participants (mean age: 26 years SD 5; mean BMI: 23.9 SD 2.7; shoe size: US 9–11) with no history of insole related condition/disorder, were tested on two separate days with a minimum of 48 hours between sessions to allow full recovery from the walking intervention. Participants were consistently scheduled at the same day time to reduce the risk of impacting their energy level and were asked to wear the same pair of running shoes during each session. Prior to testing, each participant read and signed a consent form.

Two different insole conditions were evaluated in a randomized order, including a control (i.e. no insole added, CTRL) and a SSCO with custom arch support (Custom Fit®, Dr. Scholl's®, Bayer Healthcare, LLC, Whippany, NJ, USA). The selected SSCO were built off three layers: a soft top cloth for comfort and durability, a cushion layer to disperse foot pressure and reduce shocks, and a 3D arch support dual layer to best fit the morphology of each individual's arch. For each shoe size, four different SSCOs were available with different arch support characteristics. For every participant, the best SSCO fit was selected based on weight (i.e. more or less than 170 lbs) and arch type (i.e. low, medium or high arch).

### 2.2 Anthropometrics and subjective evaluations

Upon the participant's arrival, an anthropometric evaluation was performed where variables such as height, weight, foot width and arch height were measured.

### 2.3 Baseline assessments

Prior to testing, participants were asked to fill out a questionnaire to assess the intensity of their baseline fatigue using a 0–5 Likert scale (**Table 1**).

Surface bipolar Ag-AgCI EMG electrodes (Norotrode Myotronics-Noromed Inc., Kent, WA, USA) with a diameter of 10 mm and an inter electrode spacing of 22 mm were positioned on the muscle bellies of the gastrocnemius lateralis (GL) and medialis (GM) of the right leg (**Figure 1**). To enhance signal conductivity, the corresponding skin surfaces were shaved and cleaned using abrasive tape and isopropyl wipe prior to electrode positioning. According to the SENIAM guidelines [21], each electrode was placed in the direction of the underlying muscle fibers.

Following electrode placements, each participant was placed lying prone in a horizontal position on an isokinetic dynamometer (Biodex System 4, Biodex Medical Systems, USA) with the right foot fixed to a plantarflexion attachment and the lateral malleolus aligned with the centre of rotation of the dynamometer. The EMG activity of the GL and GM muscles was recorded at 2400 Hz during two

| Fatigue Level | Description |
|---|---|
| 0 – No fatigue | No fatigue. |
| 1 – Very slightly noticeable | Legs and feet feel active but no pain. |
| 2 – Slightly noticeable | Slight fatigue and pain in legs and/or feet, but not enough to cause you to change your walking pattern. |
| 3 – Noticeable | Legs and/or feet start to feel heavy and in moderate pain, to a level where you think about changing your walking pattern to help relieve your muscles. |
| 4 – Very noticeable | Heavy legs and/or feet, and in enough pain to make you change your walking pattern because you need to relieve your muscles. |
| 5 – Extremely noticeable | Legs and feet very hard to move and in a lot of pain, to the point where you immediately want to stop walking and sit down. |

**Table 1.**
*Likert scale (0–5) used to define the level of perceived fatigue for each participant.*

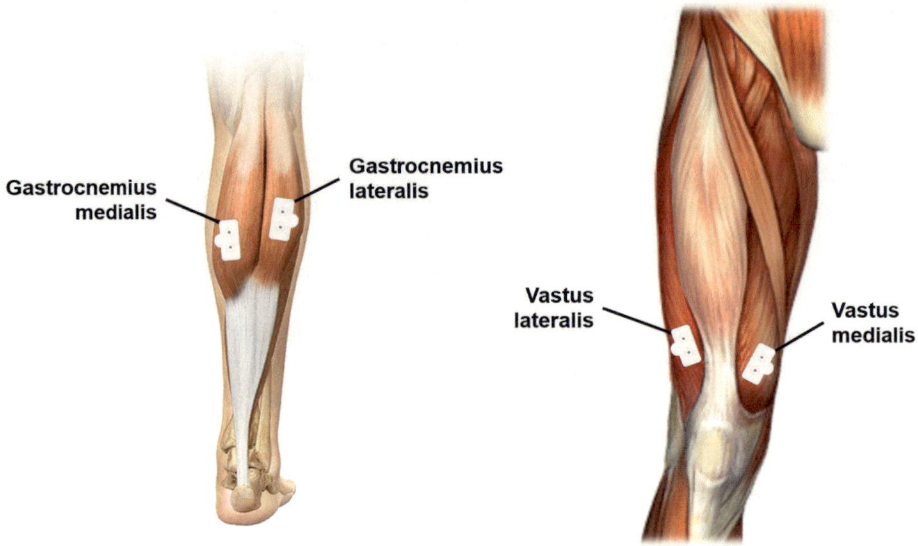


**Figure 1.**
*Left: EMG electrodes placement on the gastrocnemius lateralis (GL) and medialis (GM) - right: EMG electrodes placement on the vastus lateralis (VL) and medialis (VM).*

15-second isometric plantarflexion trials performed at 50% of the participant's maximal strength. To ensure a consistent torque output between trials and testing sessions, the maximal torque output of each subject was measured during the first day using two maximal voluntary contractions (MVC) trials. The corresponding value was then used to provide torque visual feedback during each 50% sustained contraction trials.

Participants were then asked to remove their shoes and socks and perform three 10-second standing trials and six walking trials (three steps per foot) on a foot pressure scan (Currex Footplate, Currex GmbH, Germany).

### 2.4 Walking intervention

The walking intervention was defined as a power walking trial on a 4° inclined treadmill at a constant speed of 4mph. Such settings were deemed sufficient - based on preliminary testing performed on seven volunteers - to induce fatigue in the feet and legs within a period of 30 to 60 minutes.

Prior to the intervention, additional EMG electrodes were placed on the vastus lateralis (VL) and vastus medialis (VM) (**Figure 1**). To detect heel strike, a one-dimensional (1D) accelerometer (sampling rate: 2400 Hz, encapsulated in a 20/12/5 mm plastic shell, measuring range: ± 50 g, frequency response: 0–400 Hz, mass: < 5 grams, ADXL 78, Analog Devices, Inc., Norwood, USA) was taped on the participant's right heel and synchronized with the EMG recordings.

Prior to the intervention, a 6-minute warm-up trial was performed with increasing walking speed and inclination angle (i.e. 2 minutes at 3mph and 1° incline, 2 minutes at 3.5 mph and 2.5° incline, and 2 minutes at 4mph and 4° incline). After warm-up, EMG activity of the GL, GM, VL and VM were recorded at 2400 Hz respectively for segments of 5 minutes. At the end of each segment, the participant was asked to rate his level of perceived fatigue using the same 0–5 Likert scale as the one used during the baseline assessments (**Table 1**). During the first testing session, the intervention stopped when the subject reached a fatigue level of 4 (described as heavy/sore legs and/or feet leading to voluntary changes in walking pattern to relieve muscles) on the perceived fatigue scale. The corresponding time was used to define the duration of the intervention during the second testing session. If a participant was not able to reach a fatigue level of 4 after a duration of 60 minutes or reached a fatigue level of 5 (i.e. extremely sore legs and feet very leading to the immediate need to stop the intervention), prior to 30 minutes, the intervention was stopped, and the corresponding data was not used in the analysis.

### 2.5 Post-intervention assessments

Immediately following completion of the intervention, each participant performed the same tests as describe in the baseline assessments section, starting with the foot pressure scans (standing and walking), followed by one isometric contraction trial. At the end of each session, participants were asked to rate their post-intervention perceived fatigue, as well as the comfort of the tested insoles (overall, heel, arch, forefoot).

### 2.6 Data processing

Data were all processed using custom-written Matlab codes (R2017a, MathWorks, Inc.).

#### *2.6.1 Foot pressure scans*

For each standing and walking trial performed on the foot pressure scan, the corresponding static and dynamic arch indices were calculated using the method described by, see [22], which defines the arch index as the ratio between the midfoot area (i.e. middle third of the entire footprint excluding the toes) and the area of the whole foot (toes excluded).

#### *2.6.2 EMG*

A wavelet transform using 20 non-linearly scaled wavelets (centre frequencies: 1.38, 3.86, 7.54, 12.42, 18.47, 25.69, 34.08, 43.61, 54.30, 66.12, 79.09, 93.19, 108.41, 124.76, 142.24, 160.83, 180.55, 201.37, 223.31, 246.35 Hz) was applied to the raw EMG signals recorded during each isometric contraction trials. The mean EMG frequency of each muscle was calculated using the power spectrum of the corresponding wavelet transformed signal and compared between baseline and post-intervention.

A custom-written heel-strike detection algorithm was applied to the walking EMG data to isolate each step within a defined window (i.e. 300 ms before and 600 ms after heel strike). For each step and muscle, the active portion of the EMG signal was selected using fixed time windows (i.e. from 75 ms before to 150 ms after heel strike for the GL and GM, and from 195 ms to 555 ms after heel strike for the VL and VM). The resulting active portions were then wavelet transformed using the method described above, and the corresponding power spectra were averaged for the first (non-fatigued) and last (fatigued) minute of recording.

### 2.7 Data analysis

The impact of fatigue was assessed for each variable as the relative change from non-fatigued to fatigued stages (i.e. baseline to post-intervention, first to last minute) and expressed as a percentage. A one-tailed paired T-test with alpha = 0.05 was performed to compare between insole conditions.

## 3. Results

### 3.1 Subjective fatigue assessment

A total of 21 participants reached the targeted fatigue level within 30 to 60 minutes. The remaining subjects fatigued either too quickly (N = 3) or not sufficiently (N = 6) during the intervention, and hence were not included in the analysis.

The mean absolute gain in perceived muscle fatigue was the slightly lower for the SSCO compared to the CTRL (**Table 2**). Regarding the perceived impact of each insole condition, 63% of the participants experienced improvements in foot fatigue while wearing the SSCO, and 40% experienced the same effect while wearing the CTRL.

### 3.2 Static and dynamic arch indices

The SSCO condition resulted in a slightly smaller increase in static arch index for the left foot compared to CTRL, and in a slight decrease in static and dynamic arch indices for the right foot (**Figure 2**). A strong variability was observed among subjects (i.e. large standard error) and none of the arch index results reached statistical significance (P-values >0.05, **Table 3**).

| | | CTRL | SSCO |
|---|---|---|---|
| Mean absolute gain in perceived muscle fatigue during intervention | | 3.30 | 2.98 |
| Mean intensity of perceived muscle fatigue | Baseline | 0.40 | 0.42 |
| *from 0 (no fatigue) to 5 (exhaustion)* | Post-intervention | 3.70 | 3.40 |
| Percentage of the population experiencing improvements in foot fatigue | | 40% | 63% |

**Table 2.**
*Mean absolute gain in perceived muscle fatigue (i.e. difference between baseline and post-intervention mean intensity of perceived muscle fatigue) and impact of each insole condition with respect to foot fatigue perception (N = 21).*

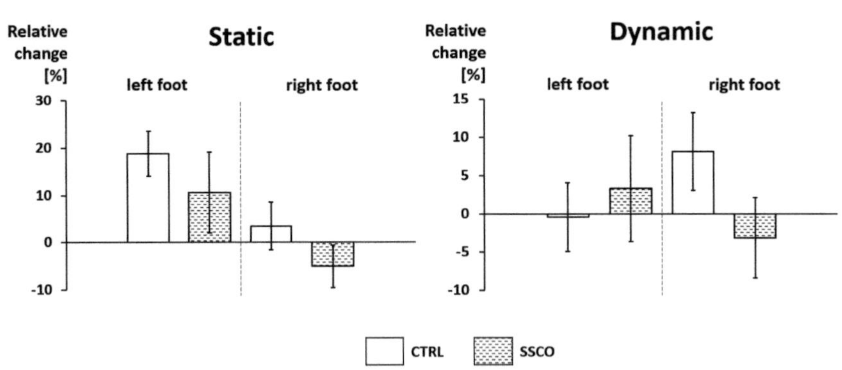


**Figure 2.**
*Mean relative change in static (left) and dynamic (right) arch index from baseline to post-intervention. The error bars represent the standard error resulting from the data of all fatigued subjects (N = 21).*

## 3.3 Mean EMG activity and frequency

### *3.3.1 50% isometric contraction*

An increase in mean EMG activity was observed in the GL and GM muscles for both insole conditions (**Figure 3**). The corresponding increases were smaller for the GL compared to the GM in the CTRL condition, while the mean EMG activity of these two muscles increased similarly when participants were wearing the SSCO. For both conditions and both muscles, the relative changes in mean EMG frequency were negligible (~1%). None of these changes reached statistical significance when comparing across conditions (**Table 3**).

| | | | CTRL | SSCO | P-value |
|---|---|---|---|---|---|
| Foot pressure scan | Static arch index | L | +19% (SE 5%) | +11% (SE 9%) | 0.14 |
| | | R | +3% (SE 5%) | −5% (SE 4%) | 0.13 |
| | Dynamic arch index | L | −0.5% (SE 5%) | +3% (SE 7%) | 0.39 |
| | | R | +8% (SE 5%) | −3% (SE 5%) | 0.10 |
| 50% isometric contraction | Mean EMG activity | GL | +13% (SE 6%) | +20% (SE 9%) | 0.29 |
| | | GM | +30% (SE 16%) | +23% (SE 9%) | 0.38 |
| | Mean EMG frequency | GL | +1% (SE 1%) | +0% (SE 1%) | 0.33 |
| | | GM | +0% (SE 1%) | +1% (SE 1%) | 0.20 |
| Uphill power walking intervention | Mean EMG activity | GL | −6% (SE 3%) | −8% (SE 2%) | 0.24 |
| | | GM | +0% (SE 2%) | −4% (SE 2%) | 0.08 |
| | | VL | +8% (SE 4%) | +5% (SE 3%) | 0.17 |
| | | VM | +1% (SE 5%) | +2% (SE 4%) | 0.45 |
| | Mean EMG frequency | GL | +6% (SE 1%) | +6% (SE 1%) | 0.39 |
| | | GM | +5% (SE 0%) | +4% (SE 1%) | 0.33 |
| | | VL | +0% (SE 2%) | +1% (SE 0%) | 0.28 |
| | | VM | +3% (SE 2%) | +1% (SE 1%) | 0.23 |

**Table 3.**
*Mean relative change in arch index (static and dynamic) and mean EMG activity and frequency (for GL and GM during 50% isometric contraction and for GL, GM, VL, VM during the uphill power walking intervention) from non-fatigued to fatigued (SE: Standard error) (N = 21).*

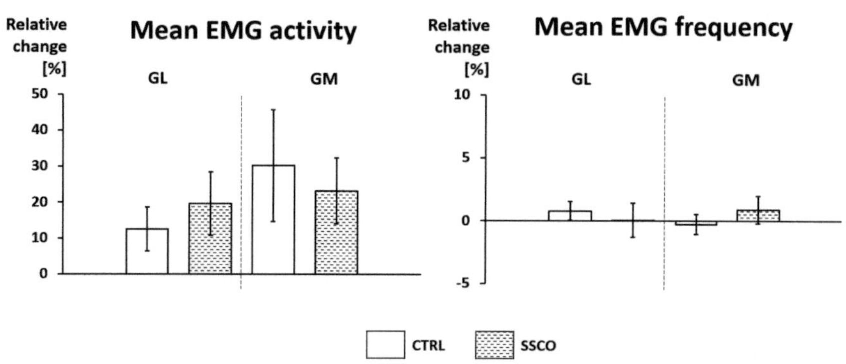


**Figure 3.**
*Mean relative change in mean EMG activity (left) and frequency (right) of the GL and GM muscles from baseline to post-intervention. The error bars represent the standard error resulting from the data of all fatigued subjects (N = 21).*

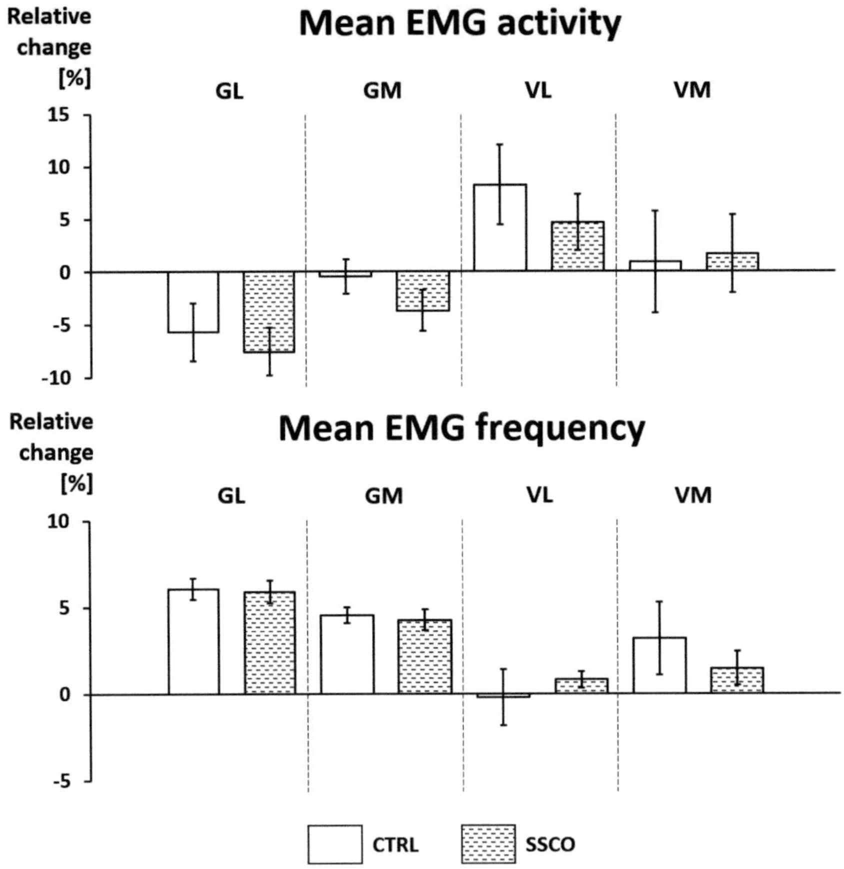


**Figure 4.**
*Mean relative change in mean EMG activity (top) and frequency (bottom) of the GL, GM, VL and VM muscles from first to last minute of the intervention. The error bars represent the standard error resulting from the data of all fatigued subjects (N = 21).*

### *3.3.2 Uphill power walking intervention*

For both conditions, the mean EMG activity of the GL and GM decreased between the first and last minute of the intervention, while the opposite trend was observed for the VL and GM (**Figure 4** top). The decrease observed in mean EMG activity for the GL and GM was slightly stronger, and the increase in mean EMG activity of the VL was slightly less for the SSCO condition compared to CTRL. No specific difference could be observed when comparing the changes in mean EMG frequency between conditions (**Figure 4** bottom). None of the results reached statistical significance when comparing across conditions (**Table 3**).

## 4. Discussion

In this study, a protocol was designed to induce perceived fatigue in the lower limbs of healthy male volunteers. A variety of qualitative and quantitative variables were collected at baseline and post-intervention to assess the impact of perceived fatigue on different metrics. Two insole conditions were assessed and compared including one control (CTRL) and one self-selected customized orthotics (SSCO). The purpose of this comparison was to evaluate the impact of short-term exposure to SSCO on the perception of lower limbs fatigue. This study was motivated by the fact that, to our knowledge, no investigation had yet presented the potential effect that this new semi-custom insole design may have on the physiology and biomechanical behavior of the lower extremities. In comparison, many reports have highlighted the benefits of customized orthotics, especially regarding their positive impact on balance [2] and pressure distribution [3, 4], which appear to reduce foot pain [1] and improve the quality of life of people with specific lower limb conditions [5–14]. As a result, this study aimed at providing new insights regarding the potential impact of wearing SSCO over a short period of time (sub-hour) on selected variables associated with foot morphology, lower limb muscle activity and perceived fatigue.

In terms of subjective assessment, most of the participants (N = 21) reached the targeted perceived fatigue level within the limited time window defined by the protocol. Among these 21 participants, the mean absolute gain in perceived muscle fatigue was slightly lower when the SSCO were worn. Considering that participants started both trials with the same level of baseline fatigue and that the duration of the intervention was constant across conditions, this indicates that the SSCO helped to slightly reduce the sensation of muscle fatigue during the intervention. In addition, 63% of these participants reported experiencing improvements in foot fatigue when wearing the SSCO. Such insights agree with, see [16], who reported that 68% of their tested population experienced improved foot fatigue after wearing customized orthotics during long periods of standing and walking.

Regarding the relative change in arch index, for both conditions, small differences were observed between left and right foot, as well as between static and dynamic trials. The largest change was found statically on the left foot, where the increase in arch index was slightly lower for the SSCO compared to CTRL. Considering that an increase in arch index indicates a flattening of the arch, such insight may indicate that the integrity of the arch of the left foot was slightly less impacted while wearing the SSCO. Knowing that SSCO were designed to provide additional arch support and if we hypothesize that a flattening of the arch is associated with fatigue (i.e. loss of muscle integrity over time), this result could potentially be linked to the findings of, see [17], who reported that insoles with custom arch support help reduce the impact of fatigue during up- and downhill walking. However, none of the results presented in the current study reached statistical significance. This could be explained by the large standard errors, which is expected to result from the morphological differences between participants (i.e. low vs. high arch). As a result, these results appear challenging to interpret and further investigations should focus on populations with similar arch types to assess whether these standard errors would be decreased.

The mean EMG activity of the GL and GM muscles calculated during the 50% isometric contraction increased between baseline and post-intervention for both conditions. If we hypothesize that the mean EMG activity reflects the number of motor units that is required to perform a certain task, this observation could indicate that, when fatigue occurs, groups of motor units lose their ability to generate a consistent amount of force, therefore leading to more motor units being recruited [23, 24]. The comparison between conditions showed a slightly lower increase in EMG activity for the GM while wearing the SSCO, indicating a potential smaller impact of fatigue on the corresponding muscle. However, the opposite trend was found for the GL during the same task. In addition, the mean EMG activity of these two muscles decreased for both conditions between the first and the last minute of the walking trial, while the opposite trend was found for the VL and VM. Considering the large standard errors and the lack of statistical significance, these findings remain challenging to interpret.

Almost no change was observed with respect to mean EMG frequency during the 50% isometric contraction. However, the mean EMG frequency of the GL and GM muscles increased between the first and last minute of the walking intervention. This indicates that the firing rate of the corresponding motor units increased with fatigue, which is the opposite of the expected behavior reported in the literature [23]. No significant change was observed in terms of mean EMG frequency for the VL and VM muscles throughout the intervention.

These results reflect the complexity of measuring and interpreting long dynamic EMG signals, which can easily be impacted by several external factors such as excessive sweating or skin motion artifacts. In addition, it should be noted that the use of EMG for fatigue assessment has been severely debated in the last few decades, mostly due to the constantly changing definition of the actual fatigue phenomenon. Fatigue was originally broadly defined as the inability to maintain a specific force [25], which became more specific later as the decrease in the force production ability of the neuromuscular system during sustained contractions [26]. Due to the limitations of such definitions with respect to protocol design (i.e. purely static [27]), the definition of fatigue has been evolving throughout the year in order to allow dynamic measurements [28]. However, the scientific community has still not settled on a standard definition of this very subjective concept and its potential assessment, which shows that further research is still needed to elaborate a reliable definition of fatigue and to design consistent protocols to measure it. Nevertheless, this study still resulted in 70% of the individuals experiencing fatigue, with many of those individuals demonstrating less perceived fatigue while wearing SSCO. As a result, the data from this study could be re-evaluated once a more reliable definition of fatigue using EMG is established.

Several limitations should be noted with respect to the design of this study. First, none of the results reached statistical significance, and therefore, every conclusion should be interpreted with care. This may be due to the fact that the sample size was small and included people with slightly different morphologies and physical condition. While all attempts were made to control for such population characteristics, they remain challenging to assess prior to recruitment (i.e. arch type, physical condition with respect to uphill power walking). As a result, large standard errors were observed, which may have been reduced if the sample size had been a bit larger. A large sample size would also have allowed the potential classification of participants based on their morphological characteristics, which should be further explored in future studies.

The short time exposure to the new insole condition (i.e. less than one hour wearing the SSCO) was also a limitation that may not have given enough time for some morphological changes to occur. Future work should inspect the potential long-term impact of wearing such orthotics on the physiological and biomechanical behavior of the lower limbs. It should also be noted that the experiment was not blinded. While participants were unaware of the design and purpose of the SSCO, it was impossible to blind them to the fact that the insoles in their shoes had been changed. To try and limit the potential testing order impact, the session order was randomized among participants.

The very subjective aspect of fatigue and the way it is defined should also be included as an important limitation. In this study, participants were given a specific definition of perceived fatigue (**Table 1**) which was designed to be as intuitive as possible but remains a purely qualitative measure. Finally, the lack of literature regarding the potential impact of SSCO on the physiological and biomechanical behavior of the lower extremities made the direct comparisons with previous studies impossible.

## 5. Conclusion

In conclusion, this study provided a preliminary framework that aimed at better understanding the physiological and biomechanical consequences of wearing SSCO. Some of the preliminary findings presented in this study indicated that wearing SSCO may have some benefits with respect to perceived fatigue, arch support, and lower limb muscle fatigue. Nevertheless, additional work should be accomplished to fully understand how this new insole design impacts the lower extremities during a more diversified range of physical activities (i.e. standing, running, etc.). In addition, future work should focus on measuring the potential long-term impact (i.e. several days, weeks, months) of such orthotics by investigating potential morphological, perceptual or biomechanical changes around multiple body segments, such as the lower back, the knees and feet.

## Acknowledgements

The authors wish to thank all the participants who accepted to be involved in this study.

## Conflict of interest

The authors declare no conflict of interest.

## Notes/thanks/other declarations

This work was supported by Bayer Healthcare, LLC (Whippany, NJ, USA). All authors were fully involved in the study and preparation of the manuscript.

## Author details

Benjamin Dourthe*, Judith Osterloh, Vinzenz Von Tscharner, Sandro Nigg and Benno M. Nigg
Human Performance Laboratory, Faculty of Kinesiology, University of Calgary, Calgary, Canada

*Address all correspondence to: benjamin.dourthe@gmail.com

## References

[1] Amer AO, Jarl GM, Hermansson LN. The effect of insoles on foot pain and daily activities. Prosthetics and Orthotics International. 2014;**38**:474-480. DOI: 10.1177/0309364613512369

[2] Shin JY, Ryu YU, Yi CW. Effects of insoles contact on static balance. Journal of Physical Therapy Science. 2016;**28**:1241-1244. DOI: 10.1589/jpts.28.1241

[3] Tsung BYS, Zhang M, Mak AFT, Wong MWN. Effectiveness of insoles on plantar pressure redistribution. Journal of Rehabilitation Research and Development. 2004;**41**:767. DOI: 10.1682/JRRD.2003.09.0139

[4] Jung J-Y, Kim J-H, Kim K, Trieu PH, Won Y-G, Kwon D-K, et al. Evaluation of insole-equipped ankle foot or thosis for effect on gait based on biomechanical analysis. Korean J Sport Biomech. 2010;**20**:469-477. DOI: 10.5103/KJSB.2010.20.4.469

[5] Mandolini M, Brunzini A, Germani M. A collaborative web-based platform for the prescription of custom-made insoles. Adv Eng Informatics. 2017;**33**:360-373. DOI: 10.1016/j.aei.2016.10.004

[6] Rathleff MS, Richter C, Brushøj C, Bencke J, Bandholm T, Holmich P, et al. Custom-made foot Orthoses decrease medial foot loading during drop jump in individuals with Patellofemoral pain. Clinical Journal of Sport Medicine. 2016;**26**:335-337. DOI: 10.1097/JSM.0000000000000262

[7] Skou ST, Hojgaard L, Simonsen OH. Customized foot insoles have a positive effect on pain, function, and quality of life in patients with medial knee osteoarthritis. Journal of the American Podiatric Medical Association. 2013;**103**:50-55. DOI: 10.7547/1030050

[8] Albert S, Rinoie C. Effect of custom orthotics on plantar pressure distribution in the pronated diabetic foot. The Journal of Foot and Ankle Surgery. 1994;**33**:598-604

[9] Postema K, Burm PE, Zande ME, Limbeek JV. Primary metatarsalgia: The influence of a custom moulded insole and a rockerbar on plantar pressure. Prosthetics and Orthotics International. 1998;**22**:35-44. DOI: 10.3109/03093649809164455

[10] Windle CM, Gregory SM, Dixon SJ. The shock attenuation characteristics of four different insoles when worn in a military boot during running and marching. Gait & Posture. 1999;**9**:31-37. DOI: 10.1016/S0966-6362(99)00002-8

[11] Kang JH, Chen M Der, Chen SC, Hsi WL. Correlations between subjective treatment responses and plantar pressure parameters of metatarsal pad treatment in metatarsalgia patients: A prospective study. BMC Musculoskeletal Disorders 2006;7:1-8. doi:10.1186/1471-2474-7-95.

[12] Mueller MJ, Lott DJ, Hastings MK, Commean PK, Smith KE, Pilgram TK. Efficacy and mechanism of orthotic devices to unload metatarsal heads in people with diabetes and a history of plantar ulcers. Physical Therapy. 2006;**86**:833-842. DOI: 10.1093/ptj/86.6.833

[13] Chantelau E, Haage P. An audit of cushioned diabetic footwear: Relation to patient compliance. Diabetic Medicine. 1994;**11**:114-116. DOI: 10.1111/j.1464-5491.1994.tb00240.x

[14] Paton JS, Stenhouse EA, Bruce G, Zahra D, Jones RB. A comparison of customised and prefabricated insoles to reduce risk factors for neuropathic

diabetic foot ulceration : a participant - blinded randomised controlled trial 2011:1-11. doi:10.1186/1757-1146-5-31.

[15] Choi JK, Cha EJ, Kim KA, Won Y, Kim JJ. Effects of custom-made insoles on idiopathic pes cavus foot during walking. Bio-medical Materials and Engineering. 2015;**26**:S705-S715. DOI: 10.3233/BME-151362

[16] Sobel E, Levitz SJ, Caselli MA, Christos PJ, Rosenblum J. The effect of customized insoles on the reduction of postwork discomfort. J Am Pod Med Assoc. 2001;**91**:515-520. DOI: 10.7547/87507315-91-10-515

[17] Huang YP, Kim K, Song CY, Chen YH, Peng H Te. How arch support insoles help persons with flatfoot on uphill and downhill walking. J Healthc Eng 2017;2017. doi:10.1155/2017/9342789.

[18] MacConaill M, Basmajian J. Muscles and movements: A basis for human kinesiology. Balt Williams Wilkins. 1977

[19] Umeki Y. Static results of medial foot arch. Nippon Seikeigeka Gakkai Zasshi. 1991;**65**:891-901

[20] Tsung BYS, Zhang M, Fan YB, Boone DA. Quantitative comparison of plantar foot shapes under different weight-bearing conditions. Journal of Rehabilitation Research and Development. 2003;**40**:517-526. DOI: 10.1682/JRRD.2003.11.0517

[21] Hermens HJ, Freriks B, Merletti R, Stegeman D, Blok J, Rau G, et al. European recommendations for surface ElectroMyoGraphy. Roessingh Res Dev. 1999:8-11. DOI: 10.1016/S1050-6411(00)00027-4

[22] Cavanagh PR, Rodgers MM. The arch index: A useful measure from footprints. Journal of Biomechanics. 1987;**20**:547-551. DOI: 10.1016/0021-9290(87)90255-7

[23] Viitasalo JHT, Komi PV. Signal characteristics of EMG during fatigue. European Journal of Applied Physiology and Occupational Physiology. 1977;**37**:111-121

[24] Marco G, Alberto B, Taian V. Physiological measurement surface EMG and muscle fatigue: Multi-channel approaches to the study of myoelectric manifestations of muscle fatigue. Inst Phys Eng Med Print UK Physiol Meas. 2017;**38**:27-60. DOI: 10.1088/1361-6579/aa60b9

[25] Edwards RH. Human muscle function and fatigue. Ciba Foundation Symposium. 1981;**82**:1-18

[26] Bigland-Ritchie B, Johansson R, Lippold OC, Woods JJ. Contractile speed and EMG changes during fatigue of sustained maximal voluntary contractions. Journal of Neurophysiology. 1983;**50**:313-324. DOI: 10.1152/jn.1983.50.1.313

[27] McComas AJ, Miller RG, Gandevia SC. Fatigue brought on by malfunction of the central and peripheral nervous systems. Advances in Experimental Medicine and Biology. 1995;**384**:495-512

[28] Enoka RM, Stuart DG. Neurobiology of muscle fatigue. Journal of Applied Physiology. 1992;**72**:1631-1648. DOI: 10.1152/jappl.1992.72.5.1631

Chapter 6

# Orthoses Development Using Modern Technologies

*Branko Štefanovič, Mária Danko, Monika Michalíková, Lucia Bednarčíková, Viktória Rajťúková, Teodor Tóth, Marianna Trebuňová, Radovan Hudák and Jozef Živčák*

## Abstract

The aim of this study was to design, manufacture and verify orthoses using innovative methods. 3D scanning, additive manufacturing and CAD/CAM software are applied during the development process. Target group of the study are subjects with insufficient gripping and manipulating functions of the arm and forearm. Positives are obtained using a hand-held 3D scanner Artec Eva. Specific 3D scanning methodology is applied during this process. Individual orthoses are designed in an open-source CAD software Meshmixer and manufactured by FDM (Fused Deposition Modeling) additive technology from a biocompatible plastic material. All models are inspected and verified in an analysis software VGStudio MAX. Given methodology can be used not only for this specific purpose, but also for orthosis development in general.

**Keywords:** orthosis, additive manufacturing, 3D scanning, CAD/CAM, fused filament fabrication

## 1. Introduction

An orthosis or orthotic device is a device applied to the body to replace lost function of locomotor systems or to help restore lost or damaged function, to stabilize or immobilize a part of the body, to improve alignment, prevent deformation, protect against injury or assist in movement, or function [1].

Orthoses are used, to:

- align or position limb segments to enhance voluntary limb movement and improve function (e.g., an ankle-foot orthosis [AFO] to provide prepositioning of the foot during swing limb advancement and stability during the stance phase of gait);
- minimize the influence of abnormal tone on posture and movement (tone-inhibiting designs);
- provide individuals with a variety of comfortable and safe positions in which they can sleep, eat, travel, work, or play;

- promote joint alignment and minimize risk of contracture development and other secondary musculoskeletal sequelae (especially in growing children);
- protect a limb following orthopedic surgery performed to correct deformity or instability;
- enhance alignment following pharmacological intervention with botulinum toxin;
- provide alternative methods for mobility [2].

These are orthopedic devices that affect the function of the musculoskeletal system: they keep body parts in the desired positions or bring them into the necessary positions, sometimes replacing lost functions, or bringing the disability to a tolerable condition. Furthermore, they are devices attached to the patient's body, which affect the condition and operation of the musculoskeletal system. This means that they do not compensate for the anatomical loss of the limb, but partially compensate for the lost function. The Committee for Prosthetic Research and Development (CPRD) categorized orthoses with respect to anatomical segments and joints. It created, firmly established and implemented a system of abbreviations derived from the first letters of the name of the orthosis in English for each category. Within the international Standards By ISO, the technical committee TC 168 has introduced the mentioned terminology, which is accepted worldwide [1, 3–5].

These devices are manufactured individually or in series production, from different materials and in different sizes according to the expected length of use and the burden also related to the patient's lifestyle. When using mass-produced orthopedic-prosthetic devices (in a sufficient size range based on the anthropometrically determined dimensions of healthy people), the choice and application of a suitable device does not pose a problem. In some cases, this device may require only minimal adjustments (e.g. adjustment of the fastening strap) during the test by a qualified person (orthopedic technician, doctor). Another case is an orthosis made to measure according to the individual requirements of the individual. The traditional production process consists of the phase of taking the necessary measurements, the phase of production of the model (gypsum positive, which is made by casting gypsum) and then the creation of an orthotic device from the required materials [1, 3].

In the final phase, it is necessary to take into account the specific physiological, kinesiological and biomechanical properties that will be placed on the orthosis, structural and material characteristics, use of joints, locks and other biomechanical elements, so that the orthosis fulfills its purpose [1, 5, 6].

The goal of an orthotic device is to help a person with a disability achieve the highest level of functional independence and integration into the community. The design, manufacture and installation of orthoses and ancillary equipment is an important part of the treatment regimen [1, 4, 7].

Of course, an orthopedic device must always be prescribed by a specialist. Because, it is an aid that acts and influences the function of the locomotor system, it can harm the patient can lead to progression of the damage. It is therefore necessary that the technician who equips the patient with orthopedic aids understands the work well and is sufficiently prepared in the field of craftsmanship.

For the technician to be able to determine the correct functional type of orthosis and its optimal design, he needs to be able to assess the overall physical condition of the patient, or the affected segment. Basic examination methods, which include manual muscle testing (MMT), range test (ROM) and sensory testing, thus provide the technician with important information for an individual design of the structure and structure of the device [1, 8–10]. This knowledge, combined with the technical skills required in the manufacturing process and installation of these devices, lead to successful outcomes for patients [1, 4, 7].

### 1.1 Materials

Depending on the type of orthosis, the location of its action, the type of treatment, a combination of different materials (metals, plastics, leather, composites, foams, rubber and other materials) is chosen. The material is often selected to achieve the desired clinical result, while guaranteeing the required technical strength and environmental resistance [3, 10].

The choice of material for a given design depends in part on an understanding of the basic principles of mechanics and materials, force concepts, deformation and failure of structures under load, improving the mechanical properties by heat treatment, the manufacturing process and also has an impact on the proper functioning of the orthotic device. Among the traditionally used materials we can mention metals (connecting materials), they are also plastics, textiles, rubbers and leather have a wide range of uses. Development of new materials, especially the possibility of using new composite materials (plastic matrix with reinforcing fibers), which provide better mechanical properties and aspects of biocompatibility [3].

When using plastics, a distinction is made between low and high temperature plastics, while their use depends mainly on the location for which the orthosis is intended and the purpose of its use. In the area of the forearm and hand, low-temperature thermoplastics are usually sufficient, which can be modeled directly on the patient's body surface after heating to the working temperature (60 to 70° C). Especially orthoses intended for the fixation of affected joints, it is suitable to use either high-temperature thermoplastics, or low-temperature thermoplastics, but with a greater thickness (3.2 mm). These types of upper limb orthoses are also produced by lamination, but they are mainly those that are intended for long-term application in permanent disabilities. Large progress is being made mainly due to the wide range of materials currently available to the orthopedic technician. The ability to produce custom devices with very complex accuracy has improved the customization of the devices. Materials with a high strength-to-weight ratio have made the equipment lighter and materials that bend smoothly have improved achievable functions and performance. Knowledge of materials helps the technician in the production process and in the use of new techniques, such as additive production. As technologies and materials are constantly advancing, it is important that the orthopedic technician is constantly informed about innovations, technological procedures and materials, so that he can provide the patient with adequate care for progress [3].

### 1.2 Fabrication

#### *1.2.1 Conventional production of orthoses*

Upper limb orthoses are manufactured using plastics, while the production of low-temperature and high-temperature thermoplastics has a significantly different technological process. With low-temperature thermoplastics, processing is faster and easier. A shape is cut from the plastic or cut out according to the choice of the orthosis, which is then heated to a temperature of 60 to 70°C (depending on the thickness of the material and its properties). The material can be heated to the operating temperature in either a water bath or by dry heating. After isolation of the patient's body, the plastic is formed directly on the limb, where the knowledge and experience of an orthopedic technician are necessary for the final position of the segment of the affected segment to be correct. Gypsum positives are used as a basis for the production of orthoses from high-temperature thermoplastics. However, before starting the plastering itself, it is necessary to fill in the measurement sheet. For an orthopedic technician, it is important to assess the range of motion in terms of mobility in a targeted way to create a design for a functional orthopedic device. Based on the initial examinations, the maximum correction position of the given segment is assessed. According to the required function of the orthosis, the maximum correction position of individual segments and its time tolerability are determined. If the joints are physiologically loaded, the properties and construction of the orthosis must not change this loading situation. When plastering in practice, plaster bandages are most often used, which are attached to the limb that will be plastered and shaped at the same time. It is important to pay attention to the load points and correct the shape before the plaster hardens. It is also very important to draw landmarks and painful areas on plastered parts of the body. When removing a plaster cast, it is very important to note and mark all bone growths (bumps) that protrude to the surface or are well palpable under the skin, as some of them are important landmarks. They are marked with a dermo-graphic pencil so that they are well pressed onto the gypsum casting. Although the casting itself is in principle accurate, if the patient moves or adjustments are not made correctly, this will affect the shape or function of the orthosis. This is the case when the skill of an orthotist is shown. With the gypsum positive finished, it is necessary to decide whether to use a high-temperature thermoplastic or to make the orthosis by lamination [5, 11].

The techniques used to make traditional metal and leather orthoses and thermoplastic orthoses have not changed. What has changed is where these devices are made and whether they are made for a specific patient or mass-production. In the search for production efficiency and cost savings, along with the limitations of established production technologies, many prosthetics manufacturers have chosen the "multi-model for all" approach. They basically create several different standardized sizes and a neutral look (in terms of color, texture, etc.). Using these so-called stencils, thousands of aids are produced every year.

Due to developments in data collection and software development, the use of computer-aided design (CAD) and computer-aided manufacturing (CAM), including additive manufacturing (AM), has increased for orthoses. At present, CAD/CAM methods are available for the smallest orthotic workplaces and can be used to speed up assembly as well as to facilitate off-site production in a specialized production center [5].

In order to achieve the optimal clinical result of the application of orthoses, it is necessary to make compromises in the field of choice of materials and individual components from which the choice of production method and assembly is derived [3, 8].

### *1.2.2 Innovations in the technological process of orthoses production*

The innovation of the technological process of making an orthosis may consist in the use of modern technologies in the collection of measurements and subsequent conventional production or in the modernization of the entire process of data obtainment or production. The innovation of the technological process of collecting measurement data consists in the use of 3D scanning and computer processing of scanned data into a 3D model, which replaces the gypsum positive and the subsequent use of subtractive or additive methods of positive production. In this way, we get the basis either for drawing high-temperature thermoplastic or for the following lamination process (conventional production). The innovation of the entire technological process of orthosis production also consists in digital sampling of measuring data (3D scanning) and subsequently a specific shape of the orthosis is designed in the relevant software, which is manufactured using additive technologies. Due to the cost of the purchase price of digital imaging equipment and subsequent subtraction or additive production, large companies provide the possibility of external design and production of aids, while the orthopedic technician takes the appropriate specified measures necessary for production. The process of obtaining measurement data for "branded", i.e. the orthoses patented by the manufacturer, has been simplified by using developed measuring tools. Their use in practice is conditioned by the training of the staff who gather these measurements and their use reduces the risk of error in production. This increases the adjustment and function of the orthoses and reduces the number of aids that need to be redesigned. Despite many advances in materials and manufacturing techniques, clinical judgment and the technical skill of the orthopedic technician in the conservative treatment of the patient remain the most important elements in creating a well-equipped, highly functional orthosis [3, 5, 10].

The modern approach to the creation of devices begins with the digitization of the human body and its parts in order to obtain input data from the patient's body for the needs of modeling an orthopedic device in CAD software, following its final production. In the hands of experts, this innovative method replaces the unpleasant and time-consuming plastering. Thanks to this technological process, it is possible to achieve greater accuracy, speed of device production, a new level of comfort for the patient and functionality for the field of ortho-prosthetics. Two techniques are used for data collection: measurement and scanning. The data is processed by a computer program that creates a three-dimensional image of the model. The technician then converts the data and image to adjust the positive model. Software tools allow the practitioner to accurately apply a wide range of adjustments, including bends, rotations, scaling, alignment, and adding pressures or reliefs [5].

Digitization brings to the system of orthopedic practice better control over the creation of the device and at the same time respects the know-how of the traditional method of production and the creativity of the orthopedic technician.

In general, digitization allows:

- non-contact, immediate and comfortable obtainment of measurement data via a 3D scanner,
- modification of the model thanks to a CAD software,
- the finished 3D model of the device can be made in an innovative way of production.

Most of the software used for the design of orthopedic aids use features such as templates and macros (pre-recorded sequences of adjustments) of selected orthosis designs, which further speed up design work and ensure consistency. Other features focus on the design of the final device, not just the positive form. The information is exported to a CAM machine, which is used to manufacture a modified positive model that will be used to make the orthosis [5].

The creation of digital models also brings other possibilities how to analyze possible problems that may arise as a result of design, choice of material and in connection with the production process. The computer definition of the product to be manufactured includes all dimensions and material [3, 10].

The production of positives by the subtraction method can be realized by means of multi-axis milling machines and robotic arms. The control of multiple milling cutters is simpler, but it is possible to produce mostly only less complicated shapes, which means that they are suitable for the production of models of the forearm, shoulder, or elbow joint, but not detailed models of the hand and fingers. There is a need to use robotic arms that can incorporate even the details of the positive. The semi-finished model for production can be gypsum or polyurethane blocks of material, of different sizes depending on the location. Polyurethane blocks are usually produced in different densities according to the purpose of subsequent use.

Although CAD/CAM production is currently widely available, high initial costs (scanner, software, milling machine, 3D printer) limit its use even in small orthopedic and prosthetic operations. This leads to the centralized production of orthotic devices, but it also brings limitations in the use of this technology. This also leads to new problems arising from the fact that the experts themselves do not have control over the actual construction of the equipment, as this is done by technicians at a remote production site [10].

A general feature of additive manufacturing (AM) methods is that the production is not carried out by removing the material as in a milling machining, but by gradually adding the material in the form of powder or melt in small layers. The basic principle of 3D printing is that the computer interpretation of the object serves as a direct input to the 3D printer, which creates the required physical object without special tools [12].

Thanks to AM, it is possible to produce such products that are otherwise unusable, or their price would be very high. For parts manufactured by AM, the complexity is not what the final price is based on, it is mainly based on the material used and its properties and accuracy of 3D printing. The second big advantage is production without molds and tools. The third advantage is the possibility of production from demanding, problematic materials.

There are several ways of 3D printing, which differ in technology, materials used, print speed, accuracy and strength of products or price.

At present, various 3D printing technologies are available, with material extrusion and SLS technology having the greatest application and use in the field of prosthetics and orthotics.

FDM (Fused deposition modeling) is the most common and widely used 3D printing technology today. It is an extrusion 3D printing, in which models and prototypes are formed by layering step by step from various non-toxic thermoplastic materials. The plastic fiber is guided to the printer head, where it is melted and applied in layers that gradually solidify.

The material used in the SLS (selective laser sintering) and SLM (selective laser melting) printing methods is in the form of a powder (plastic, metal, ceramic or glass powder). The printer applies a layer of powder material to the substrate by means of a built-in roller, over which a laser (for example a laser based on carbon dioxide) moves, which selectively welds it into the lower layer. Subsequently, the roller applies another layer of material until a complete 3D model is created. The resulting models are characterized by high strength.

Orthoses made with additive technologies require postprocessing, which most often consists of surface treatment (roughness, appearance, polishing, painting, painting, etc.), which differs depending on the technology used. With FDM technology, it is advised to smooth out the layers that remain present to the print to a greater or lesser extent. The need for postprocessing in the case of SLS printing is significantly reduced compared to FDM technology.

## 2. Method

### 2.1 Modern method

Mohammed et al. [13] reported that 3D scanning method of positives obtainment and CAD design of splints is quicker, non-invasive and provides greater accuracy in reproduction. On the other hand, they also report that AM splint requires longer fabrication time, which is still acceptable but less than desirable with respect to it potentially meaning an additional visitation by a potential patient. The disadvantage of longer production time is also reported by Buonamici et al. [14], however, they suggest the adoption of modern method due to the incredible benefits in terms of weight, expected comfort, breathability and the possibility of washing the immobilized segment. Barios-Muriel et al. [15], Fitzpatrick et al. [16] and Chen et al. [17] also support this theory. Li et al. [18] proposed a splint design method, which reduces the duration of the modeling phase and reduces the manufacturing phase by using multiple 3D printers to produce individual parts of the orthosis. When comparing production costs of orthoses produced by AM or conventionally, in an analysis done by Fernandez-Vincente et al. [19] the cost of AM thumb orthoses is reduced by a half compared to the traditional method of production. When producing larger orthotic devices, Redaelli et al. [20] reported that the AM fabrication of back braces can provide a valid alternative to the current fabrication methods. The overall production time from initial scanning to delivery to the patient took approximately a full working day, similarly to what is required by the thermoforming process. However, the total man-hours are reduced because of the minimal supervision necessary during the 3D printing. The cost of the AM back brace is therefore competitive compared to the production cost of a thermoformed back brace, that typically ranges from 250 to 500 euros due to the long labor time. Also, Hale et al. [21] found out that scanning to delivery of an individual AM neck brace, which takes approximately 6 weeks to produce by the traditional way, was approximately 72 hours, and the production costs of both methods is comparable.

These facts confirm the practical application of modern methods in orthoses production. The goal of this study is to apply these modern methods in the production of individual arm and forearm orthoses and propose a methodology.

### 2.2 Positives obtaining

3D scanning technology, specifically the Artec Eva (Artec 3D, Luxembourg, Luxembourg) handheld scanner, was used to create the positive of the patient's upper limb segment. A handheld scanner is a device that constantly creates images of an object by creating real-time images of the scanned object in the software of the given scanner. Using this modern method of data acquisition, we can generate a 3D model of the patient's body segment, for which an orthosis will be designed. One of the advantages of a handheld 3D scanner is that the device is compact, lightweight, portable and requires only 1 person and a laptop to operate.

The subjects′ arm and forearm were scanned with the entire upper limb being abducted with 30° rotation in the shoulder joint and 100° flexion in the elbow joint, with the thumb in opposition to the fingers and wrists at a 10° to 20° extension, and the elbow placed on a table for better support (**Figure 1**). All subjects had sufficient strength to hold the segment in position for the time which the area of interest was scanned. The scanning frequency was set to 8fps (frames per second) and no errors occurred during the positives obtaining. For this experiment, as seen in **Figure 2**, the arm and forearm of 10 adult subjects were scanned and processed.

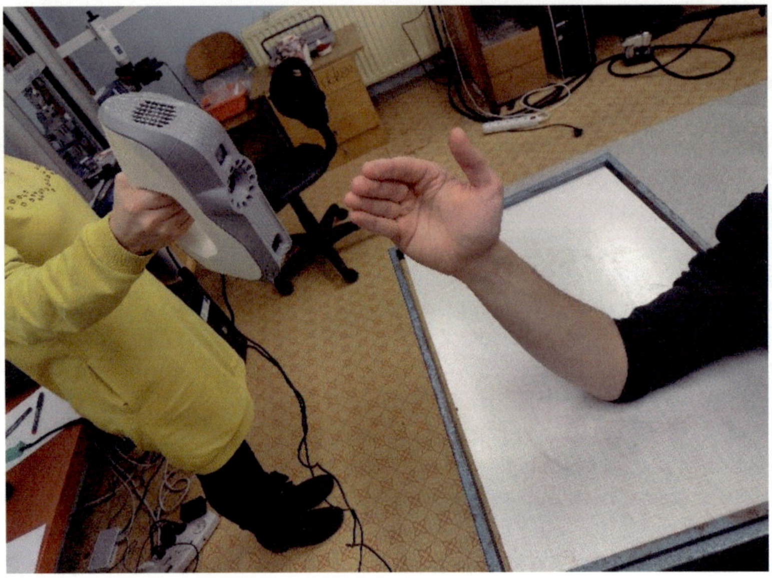

**Figure 1.**
*Arm and forearm scanning process.*

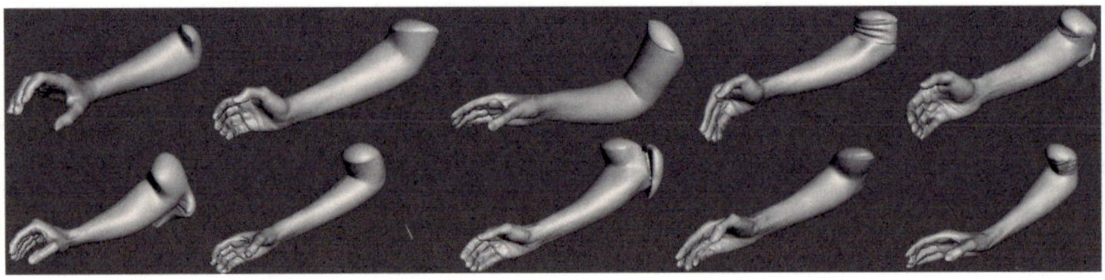

**Figure 2.**
*Obtained models of 3D scans.*

## 2.3 Orthoses 3D modeling

The Autodesk Meshmixer (Autodesk, Inc., San Rafael, CA, USA) software was used to create a digital model of the orthosis. It is a freely available modeling software in which it is possible to create and edit 3D objects. The shape of the device was sketched directly on a 3D model of a patient's upper limb segment, which we obtained by 3D scanning. When creating the contour of the device, we had to consider the coverage of the area of the segment sufficient for the orthosis to secure the wrist, thumb and the overall attachment of the device to the forearm.

The sketch of the orthosis' surface was then copied and placed on the 3D positive to create a 0.5 mm gap between the device and the area of interest. The creation of such a gap, or "offset", is important so that after the application of a real device to a given segment, there is no surface pressure, which would result in negative effects on the patient's upper limb. We can correct the size of the gap regarding whether a bio-compatible lining, which eliminates skin irritation, will be applied to the orthosis (**Figure 3**).

After creating a copy of the orthosis surface and applying the offset, the material thickness was set. Thickness of 2 mm was chosen when designing the orthosis. The thickness and choice of material is important in terms of strength and flexibility to avoid damage during use and repeated application to the given segment.

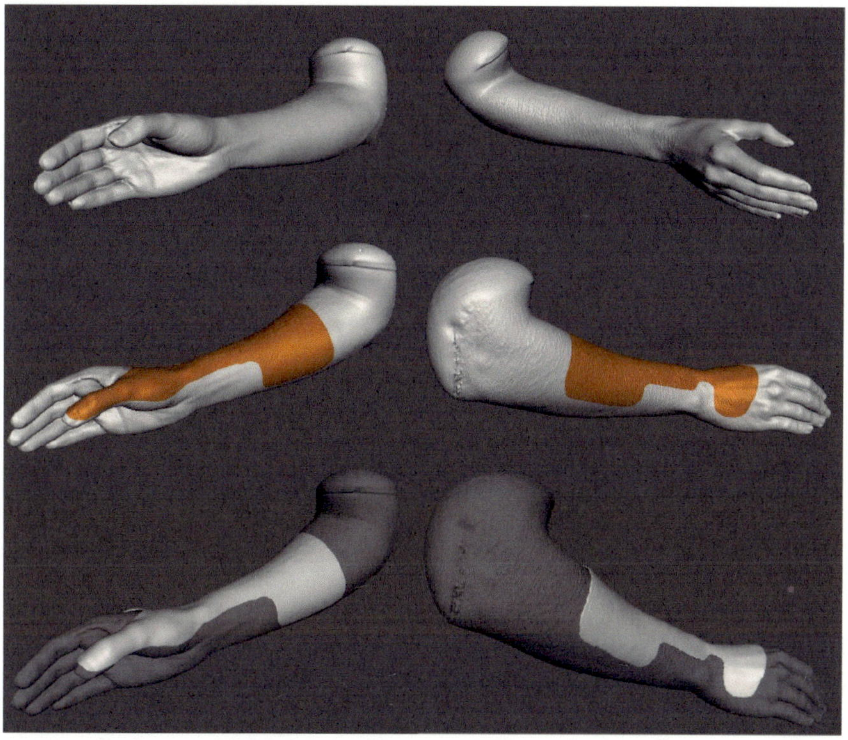

**Figure 3.**
*Orthoses design process.*

In the last step, the surface and edges of the model were smoothened, and the design of the final model was revised. Ten individual orthoses were designed and produced using FDM additive manufacturing technology.

### 2.4 Orthoses additive manufacturing

All models were manufactured on the Fortus 450mc (Stratasys Ltd., Rehotov, Israel) professional 3D printer using ABS-M30i bio-compatible polymer with a T16 tip and SR-30 support material with a T12SR30 tip. Since this printer has pre-set printing parameters for individual materials, the settings were not edited. Printing settings are listed in **Table 1**.

All models were printed one-by-one and positioned on the removable printing plate, which is stuck on the printer bed with the dorsal side oriented on the bottom (**Figure 4**).

After the manufacturing process, the printing plate was removed from the printer, all orthoses have been manually extracted and the support structures have

| Slice height | 0,010 mm |
|---|---|
| Infill | 100% |
| Part interior style | Solid |
| Visible surface | Normal |
| Support style | Box |

**Table 1.**
*Printing settings.*

been thoroughly removed. Final orthoses, as seen in **Figure 5**, have not been post processed chemically, or sand blasted.

### 2.5 Orthoses 3D scanning

All orthoses were 3D scanned in order to compare them to their actual 3D models. The Artec Eva scanner was used for this process. Individual orthoses have been fixed in a clamp by their proximal end and positioned vertically in order to capture the external and internal surface of the models (**Figure 6**).

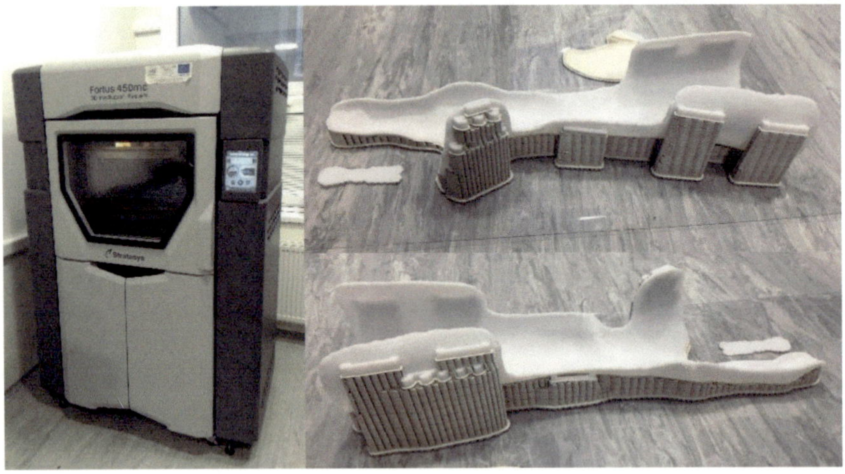


**Figure 4.**
*Fortus 450mc 3D printer (left) and an example of an orthoses manufactured by this machine (right).*

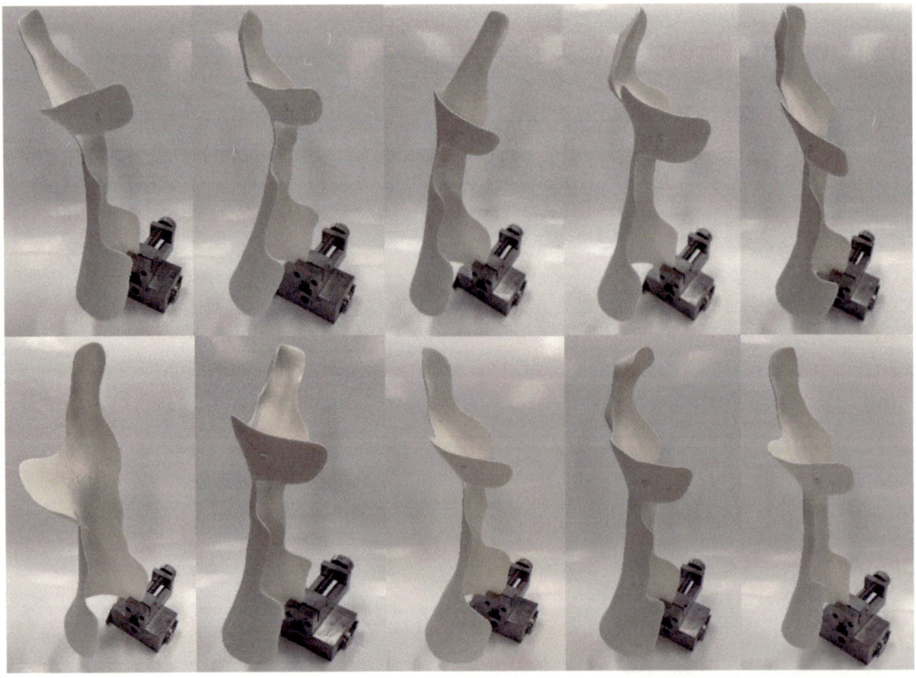

**Figure 5.**
*Final orthoses.*

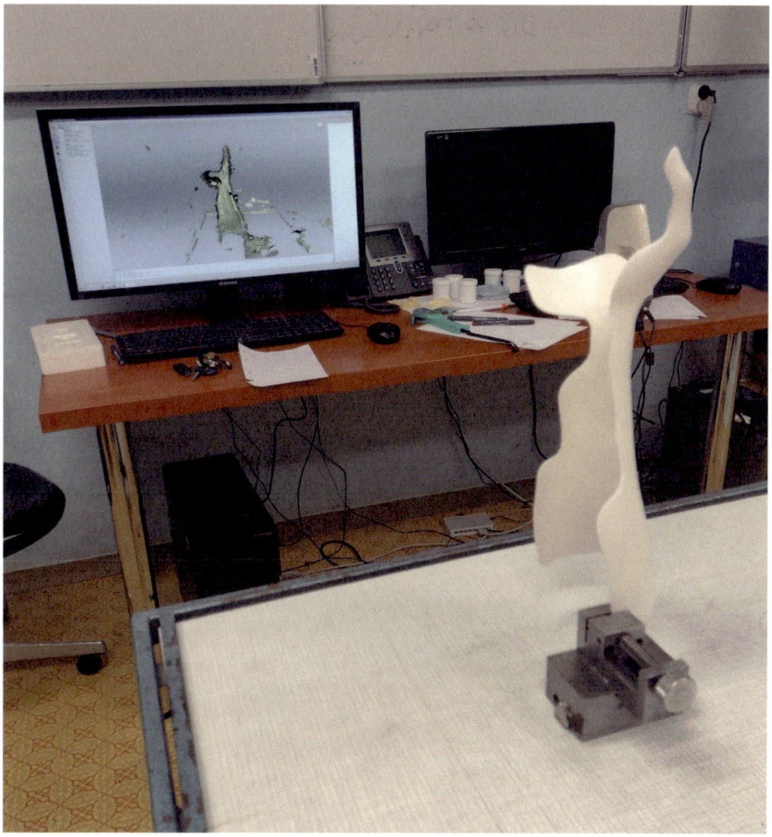

**Figure 6.**
*3D scanning of the final orthoses.*

The scanning frequency was set to 8 fps (frames per second) and no errors occurred during the positives obtaining. Scanning of 1 orthosis took approximately 10 minutes, where the scanning took approximately 5 minutes and the postprocessing of the acquired data also 5 minutes. While postprocessing the acquired data in Artec Studio13 (Artec 3D, Luxembourg, Luxembourg), artifacts surrounding the 3D scan have been constantly generating when fixing the holes in the scan. To eliminate these defects, hole filling in the software has been disabled and the scan processing has been finished in Meshmixer software, where the scans were converted to solid models (**Figure 7**).

The edges of individual models have not been smoothened to preserve the generated shape. After the finalization, all 3D models of the scans were compared to their actual STL models in VGStudio MAX (Volume Graphics, Germany) software.

### 2.6 Actual to nominal 3D model comparison

When comparing actual to nominal models we must first determine what models we are comparing. The first step was to find out if there is a difference between the models generated from the 3D scanner software and digitally solidified 3D scan models. One of these 2 models was then chosen as the actual model. These models of the orthoses were then compared to their nominal models, which are the original orthoses models designed in Autodesk Meshmixer. After the actual to nominal model comparison, the thickness of the orthoses was also verified.

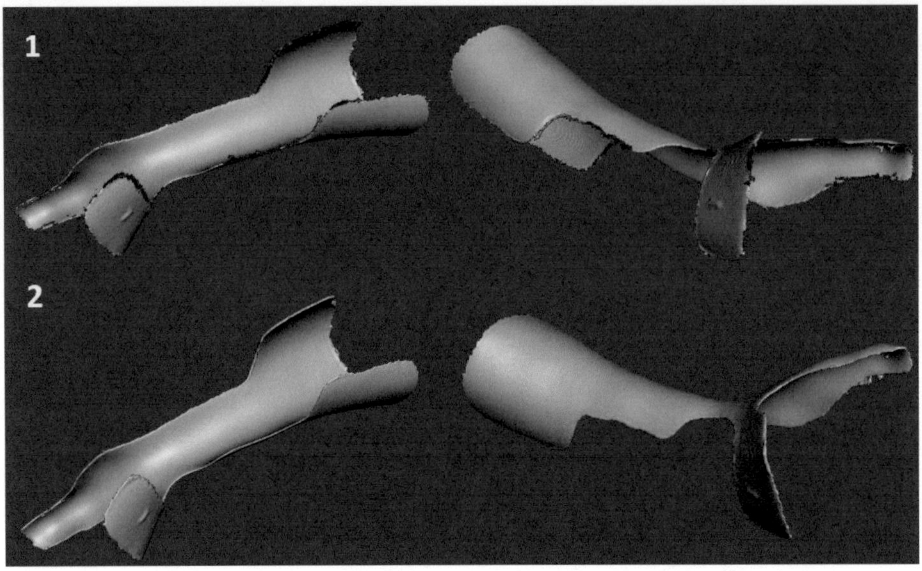


**Figure 7.**
*Model of the scan generated from Artec Studio13 (1) and solidified 3D model of the scan (2).*

# 3. Results

## 3.1 Time and material consumption

As a result, an orthosis design methodology is proposed. Time consumption of individual steps of this process has been recorder to calculate the average length of orthosis production by modern technologies.

Overall duration of the scanning and data postprocessing of individual subjects is summarized in **Table 2**. Based on these results the average duration of the arm and forearm scanning is 2 minutes and 20 seconds, and the duration of data postprocessing is 5 minutes and 20 seconds. While scanning the area of interest no complications and errors have occurred. All collected data has satisfactory quality of the surface necessary for orthosis design.

| Subject | Scanning (mm:ss) | Postprocessing (mm:ss) |
|---|---|---|
| Subject 1 | 02:49 | 05:50 |
| Subject 2 | 02:30 | 05:23 |
| Subject 3 | 02:36 | 05:32 |
| Subject 4 | 02:27 | 05:33 |
| Subject 5 | 02:15 | 05:47 |
| Subject 6 | 02:21 | 05:12 |
| Subject 7 | 02:02 | 05:05 |
| Subject 8 | 02:12 | 04:49 |
| Subject 9 | 02:05 | 05:09 |
| Subject 10 | 02:09 | 04:58 |
| **Average time** | **02:20** | **05:20** |

**Table 2.**
*Subject scanning and data postprocessing duration.*

No extra modifications of the scan 3D models were necessary during the orthosis design phase. Thanks to this fact, the design process of orthoses took approximately 3 minutes. Design duration for each orthosis is summarized in **Table 3**.

When positioning individual orthoses models on the virtual building platform of the 3D printer, the software automatically calculates the volume of the used model material, support material and the overall time of production. Average volume of model material used for the orthosis production is 65,94 $cm^3$, 57,40 $cm^3$ of support material and the average time of production is 5 hours and 18 minutes. These data are summarized in **Table 4**.

### 3.2 Verification results

The results of comparing models generated from the 3D scanner software and digitally solidified 3D scan models shows that from the deviation in the range of ±0.050 mm the models are identical. Only differences are on the edges of the

| Orthosis model | Design duration (mm:ss) |
|---|---|
| Orthosis 1 | 03:12 |
| Orthosis 2 | 03:20 |
| Orthosis 3 | 03:05 |
| Orthosis 4 | 02:58 |
| Orthosis 5 | 02:52 |
| Orthosis 6 | 03:13 |
| Orthosis 7 | 03:07 |
| Orthosis 8 | 02:53 |
| Orthosis 9 | 03:23 |
| Orthosis 10 | 03:16 |
| **Average time** | **03:11** |

**Table 3.**
*Orthoses design duration.*

| Orthosis | Model ($cm^3$) | Support ($cm^3$) | Time (hh:mm) |
|---|---|---|---|
| Orthosis 1 | 60.91 | 65.33 | 05:22 |
| Orthosis 2 | 55.23 | 50.43 | 04:58 |
| Orthosis 3 | 63.25 | 34.60 | 04:30 |
| Orthosis 4 | 72.87 | 70.33 | 06:31 |
| Orthosis 5 | 70.85 | 63.29 | 05:37 |
| Orthosis 6 | 77.58 | 71.48 | 05:56 |
| Orthosis 7 | 58.56 | 59.67 | 05:05 |
| Orthosis 8 | 69.47 | 49.41 | 05:03 |
| Orthosis 9 | 75.67 | 61.74 | 05:51 |
| Orthosis 10 | 55.04 | 47.68 | 04:25 |
| **Average value** | **65.94** | **57.40** | **05:18** |

**Table 4.**
*Orthoses printing parameters.*

models. An example is shown in **Figure 8**. Digitally solidified scan models were chosen for the actual to nominal comparison.

In **Table 5** the average deviation of solidified scan models to actual scanned models are summarized. To evaluate the differences between the actual scan model and the solidified model, the maximum deviations for 75%, 90% and 95% surface coverage were determined. These data indicate that for e.g. 95% of all values are the maximum deviation. By the deviation values of Orthosis 4 all comparisons have a deviation of less than 0.01 mm at 75% coverage, so there are only minimal changes compared to the actual model. At 90% this value is less than 0.03 mm and at 95% less than 0.08 mm. In these cases, the sets of deviations are already affected mainly by deviations caused by the closing of edges of the solidified model and possible defects.

When designing orthoses, the wall thickness was set to 2 mm. The actual thickness was measured in the "Wall thickness module" of VGStudio MAX. As a result of the analysis, the actual values range from 2.006 mm to 2.097 mm and the standard deviation is less than 0.24 mm (**Table 6**).

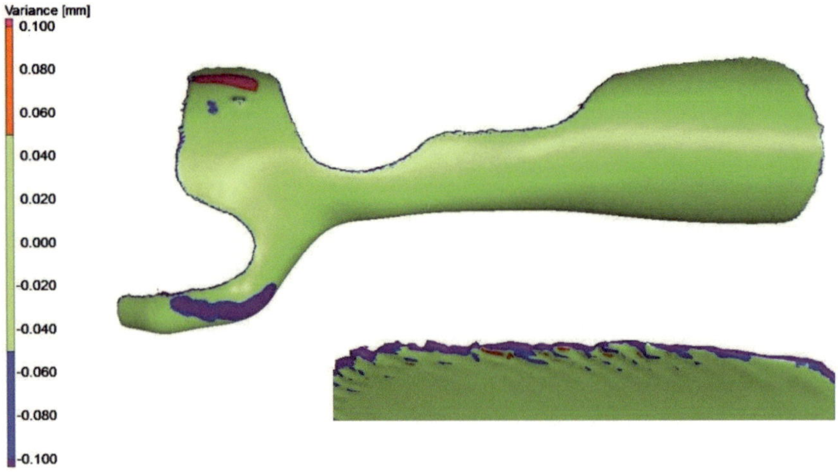


**Figure 8.**
*Original scan model and solidified scan model comparison with a detail on the edge of the model.*

| Orthosis model | Average deviation [mm] | 75% deviation [mm] | 90% deviation [mm] | 95% deviation [mm] |
|---|---|---|---|---|
| Orthosis 1 | −0.0110 | 0.0058 | 0.0131 | 0.0319 |
| Orthosis 2 | −0.0120 | 0.0059 | 0.0129 | 0.0290 |
| Orthosis 3 | −0.0110 | 0.0063 | 0.0124 | 0.0345 |
| Orthosis 4 | −0.0057 | 0.0078 | 0.0286 | 0.0793 |
| Orthosis 5 | −0.0110 | 0.0068 | 0.0132 | 0.0300 |
| Orthosis 6 | −0.0075 | 0.0059 | 0.0128 | 0.0290 |
| Orthosis 7 | −0.0098 | 0.0057 | 0.0120 | 0.0317 |
| Orthosis 8 | −0.0097 | 0.0076 | 0.0194 | 0.0527 |
| Orthosis 9 | −0.0095 | 0.0063 | 0.0153 | 0.0362 |
| Orthosis 10 | −0.0096 | 0.0052 | 0.0103 | 0.0284 |
| **Average value** | **-0.0097** | **0.0063** | **0.015** | **0.0383** |

**Table 5.**
*Average variation values of solidified scan models to actual scanned models.*

| Solidified orthosis model | Average [mm] | Standard deviation [mm] |
|---|---|---|
| Orthosis 1 | 2.031 | 0.190 |
| Orthosis 2 | 2.042 | 0.134 |
| Orthosis 3 | 2.040 | 0.224 |
| Orthosis 4 | 2.054 | 0.231 |
| Orthosis 5 | 2.065 | 0.196 |
| Orthosis 6 | 2.006 | 0.157 |
| Orthosis 7 | 2.027 | 0.163 |
| Orthosis 8 | 2.097 | 0.234 |
| Orthosis 9 | 2.082 | 0.154 |
| Orthosis 10 | 2.047 | 0.174 |
| **Average value** | **2.049** | **0.186** |

**Table 6.**
*Actual wall thickness values.*

When the scan model is compared with the actual orthosis model, it is necessary to perform their mutual alignment before performing the analyzes, as the scanned orthosis has a different coordinate system than the designed model created in the Meshmixer software. Due to the shape of the orthosis (absence of planes and simple shapes such as cylinders, etc.), their mutual alignment is possible using the Best-fit and RPS methods (reference positioning system). When using the RPS method, the Best-fit of the objects is the first step, and second the subsequent transfer of points to the current model (orthosis scan), after which the alignment itself is performed. The **Figure 9** shows an example for Best-fit alignment and RPS alignment. The figure above compares the scan of the orthosis to the solid model using the Best-fit method and below using the RPS method.

**Figure 10** shows the deviations between the two methods of alignment. It can be seen from the histogram (**Figure 11**) that the deviations are almost symmetrical with respect to zero, i.e. the two alignments are rotated relative to each other, which can also be seen in the figure.

Significant differences in models (orthosis shape) do not allow the distribution points to be distributed on all orthoses in the same way. To eliminate the effect of point placement for RPS alignment, the orthosis scan model and actual model were aligned with each other using the Best-fit method.

**Table 7** shows the data for the average deviation of the original individual orthoses model with respect to the solidified model. To evaluate the differences between the solidified scan model and the original orthosis model, the average deviation value and the maximum deviations for 90% and 95% surface coverage were determined. The average value of the deviation is close to zero and thus the distribution of deviations has the character of a normal (Gaussian) distribution. The average value for 95% coverage is 0.419 mm and 95% coverage 0.576 mm.

To control the quality of production, the thickness of the orthosis over its entire surface was also evaluated. The results in **Table 8** show that the average thickness is 1.956 mm and the standard average deviation is 0.206 mm. Compared to the nominal solidified model, the average wall thickness of the actual manufactured orthosis is smaller by 0.0931 mm and the value of the standard deviation is greater by 0.0203 mm, which are negligible differences.

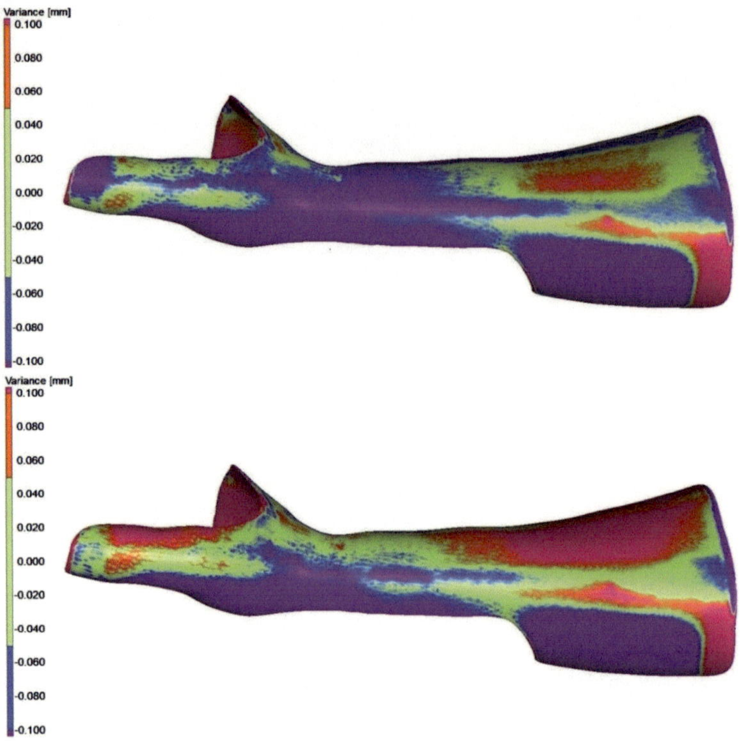


**Figure 9.**
*Best-fit alignment (up) and RPS alignment (down).*

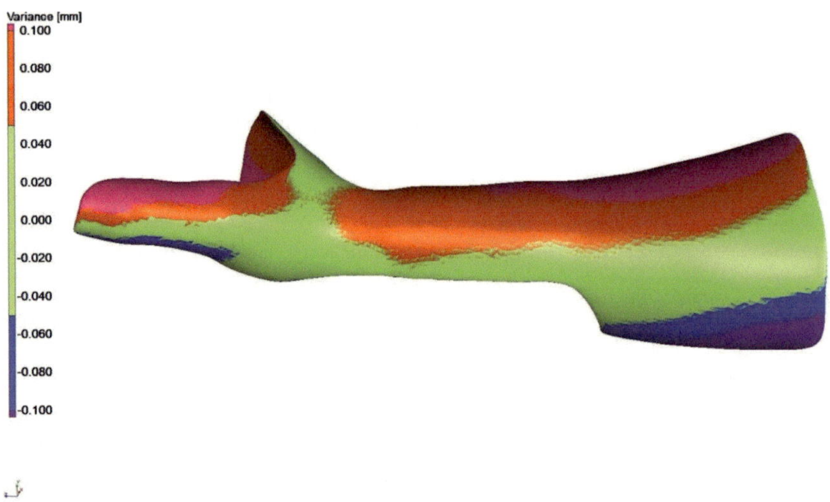


**Figure 10.**
*Deviation between the best-fit and the RPS alignment.*

Duration of the inspection and verification process has not been recorded, since it is not a part of the design methodology. Only the results of this process are relevant.

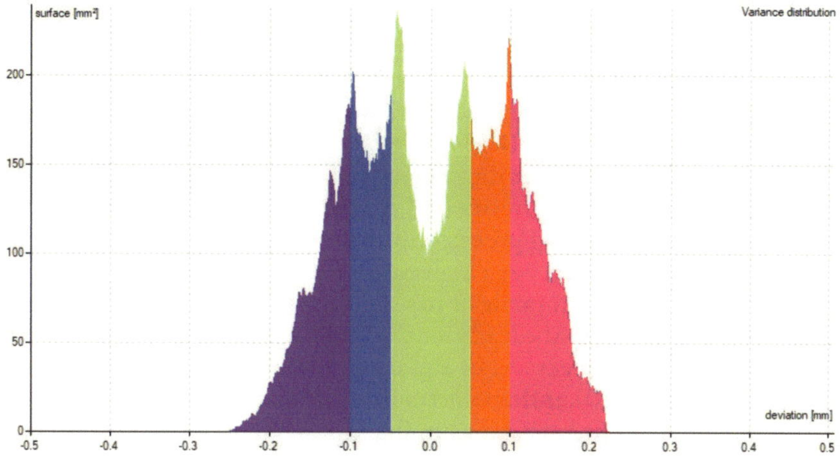


**Figure 11.**
*Histogram representing the deviations of the 2 alignment methods.*

| Orthosis | Average deviation [mm] | 90% deviation [mm] | 95% deviation [mm] |
|---|---|---|---|
| Orthosis 1 | 0.006 | 0.69 | 0.86 |
| Orthosis 2 | 0.013 | 0.24 | 0.33 |
| Orthosis 3 | 0.037 | 0.26 | 0.38 |
| Orthosis 4 | 0.026 | 0.30 | 0.46 |
| Orthosis 5 | 0.011 | 0.73 | 0.90 |
| Orthosis 6 | −0.001 | 0.46 | 0.57 |
| Orthosis 7 | 0.022 | 0.15 | 0.22 |
| Orthosis 8 | −0.014 | 0.81 | 1.25 |
| Orthosis 9 | 0.041 | 0.32 | 0.43 |
| Orthosis 10 | 0.033 | 0.23 | 0.36 |
| **Average value** | **0.017** | **0.419** | **0.576** |

**Table 7.**
*Average deviations of the original model to the solidified scan model.*

| Orthosis | Average [mm] | Standard deviation [mm] |
|---|---|---|
| Orthosis 1 | 1.95 | 0.20 |
| Orthosis 2 | 1.95 | 0.13 |
| Orthosis 3 | 1.94 | 0.27 |
| Orthosis 4 | 1.94 | 0.27 |
| Orthosis 5 | 1.97 | 0.19 |
| Orthosis 6 | 1.97 | 0.18 |
| Orthosis 7 | 1.97 | 0.18 |
| Orthosis 8 | 1.93 | 0.28 |
| Orthosis 9 | 1.97 | 0.17 |
| Orthosis 10 | 1.97 | 0.19 |
| **Average value** | **1.956** | **0.206** |

**Table 8.**
*Average thickness values of the orthoses surface.*

## 4. Discussion

When developing custom orthoses by modern technologies it is necessary to follow the steps of the method proposed in this study. First important step is the positive obtainment. Method of 3D scanning has shown to be very practical, fast, clean, precise and comfortable for the subject and the scanning staff. Working with a handheld 3D scanner is very intuitive and simple. Only 1 person and a laptop or a PC is required for the scanning process. Since the scanner is portable, it is not necessary that the subject must be in a special work environment. This fact is very important, if the subject is immobile or has movement difficulties and it's a great advantage when compared to the traditional plastering method. The positives obtainment with the postprocessing of the acquired data took less than 10 minutes average, which is much quicker than the traditional way.

Body segment positioning before scanning is important. It is necessary to stabilize the segment of interest in order to capture the desired shape. It depends on what physical health the subject is in. If the subjects have movement restrictions or have weak body strength, it is important to provide them some form of support or stabilize the scanned body segment with the help of an assistant. The assistant can help stabilize the subject, but must support the areas, which are not important for orthosis development. When scanning subjects with no movement or force limitations it is still helpful to give them some type of support, for example, in this study the subjects had their elbow joint resting on a desk, while the arm and forearm had been scanned.

Artec Eva 3D scanner, which has been used in this study is an expensive, professional scanner used mainly for scanning larger objects and structures in mechanical, design, architectural, automotive and similar industries. Nevertheless, it is also applicable in prosthetics and orthotics. In one of our studies [22], we concluded that a high-end 3D scanner is not necessary and that low-cost scanners can capture important body segments with sufficient precision for orthosis development.

Capturing the segment in its correct shape is mandatory when designing an orthotic device. If the scanned model has defects, deformities or other artifacts it cannot be used as a positive. The original model must be clean and precise so that there's no editing needed. If the 3D model of the scan is edited, it could end up in a difference between the surface of the orthosis and the body surface, which would lead to an incorrectly designed aid.

One of the objectives was to use an open-source 3D modeling software. We chose Autodesk Meshmixer, as it has functions suited to prosthesis and orthosis design. In a few easy steps it is possible to design simple orthoses suited for additive manufacturing. The design process of an arm and forearm orthosis in this software took less than 4 minutes. The interface is very clear and organized and the user does not need any special training. However, when designing medical devices, it is necessary that a skilled prosthetist operates the software. Main disadvantage of the software is that it does not have medical certification, so the models should be used only for educational and research purposes.

Choosing the correct material for the production is important from the point of manufacturing and application. Since the orthoses are meant to fix and stabilize the arm and forearm and skin contact is unavoidable, the used material needs to be strong and biocompatible. Also, the Fortus 450mc printer uses cartridges of materials suited only for this type of printer, so the range of materials is limited by the manufacturer. For these reasons the ABS-M30i has been chosen as the most suitable material. Other materials like PETG or PLA can be used for orthosis production [20], but since this 3D printer does not support these materials, they were not chosen for this study.

All models have been positioned with the dorsal side facing the printer bed. The meaning of this was to avoid support generation on the inner shell of the models to minimize support material volume and reduce postprocessing difficulty. Support structures on the inner shell could also deform the surface during the production process. From the results of the nominal to actual comparison of some models it is clear that the parts of the models that arch above the inner shell have deformed during printing. For this reason, it is advised to put support structures even on the inner shell of the models to avoid deformation.

The maximum time length of an arm and forearm orthosis produced by high or low-temperature thermoforming set by the public insurance company in Slovakia is 5 and a half man-hours. The manufacturing of a single 3D-printed individual orthosis took less than 5 and a half hours. When we add the average time of actual labor, which was approximately only 10 to 15 minutes, the whole process took less than 6 hours, which is the approximate time of an orthosis production by conventional methods for a single patient. This means, that by using proposed innovative methods, the technician can save time and design other orthotic devices, while the previous ones are producing. This time length can vary depending on the technologies used in single steps, or the number of models being developed. Duration of conventional and proposed production of arm and forearm splints is summarized in **Table 9**.

From the results of the analysis we can see that the difference between the produced orthosis and the 3D model is negligible from the point of view of orthotic application. After postprocessing and application of straps and maybe lining, these orthoses are fully functional and ready to use.

Since the manufacturing technology used in this study is a high-end, professional 3D printer, it is possibl e for hospitals, or prosthetic workshops, to produce their orthoses externally. Price of 1 orthosis, considering the material and applied technology, is approximately 70 euros. The maximum cost of an arm and forearm orthosis produced by high or low-temperature thermoforming set by the public insurance company in Slovakia is 166 euros (including materials, technology and man-hours). This means that there is a 96-euro gap between the conventional orthosis price and the 3D-printed orthosis manufacturing cost. This gap can be used to compensate the scanning, designing process and labor payment. Cost of conventional and proposed production of arm and forearm splints is summarized in **Table 9**.

If these institutions can acquire their own low-cost 3D scanner and maybe a 3D modeling software, the development process is faster, simpler and more practical, which means that the amount of produced individual orthotic devices grows. This is a favorable state not only for these institutions, but mainly for the patients themselves.

The proposed methodology, which contains orthoses design and additive manufacturing, is an adequate method for orthoses production. This method could also be used for design and manufacturing of individual prosthetic sockets for lower or upper limb prosthesis, trunk orthoses, orthotic seating systems and disability aids.

| Method | Duration (hh:mm) | Cost (euro) |
|---|---|---|
| Conventional | 05:30 | 166.00 |
| Proposed (modern) | 05:28 | 70.00 |

**Table 9.**
*Production duration and cost of conventional and modern arm and forearm orthoses.*

## 5. Conclusions

An orthoses development methodology using modern technologies has been proposed. Whole process consists of positives obtainment using a 3D scanner, orthosis design in a 3D modeling software and production using additive manufacturing technology. This methodology has been analyzed and verified by reverse engineering in an adequate software with data obtained by a proper 3D scanning device. In conclusion, it can be stated, that the proposed methodology is suitable for the use in orthotic practice.

In the future, it is planned to compare different results gained by applying other types of 3D scanners and 3D printers in the development process. The use of different types of materials is also possible if other 3D printers are used. Orthoses manufactured from different types of materials can be mechanically tested to determine, which material is most suitable for this application.

## Acknowledgements

The present article was elaborated under the support received from the project APVV-19-0290, KEGA 041TUKE-4/2019, KEGA 023TUKE-4/2020 and Stimulus for research and development 12/2018-2112/2021.

## Conflict of interest

All authors declare no conflict of interest.

## Author details

Branko Štefanovič*, Mária Danko, Monika Michalíková, Lucia Bednarčíková, Viktória Rajťúková, Teodor Tóth, Marianna Trebuňová, Radovan Hudák and Jozef Živčák
Faculty of Mechanical Engineering, Technical University of Košice, Košice, Slovakia

*Address all correspondence to: branko.stefanovic@tuke.sk

## References

[1] Yamane A. Orthotic Prescription. In: Atlas of Orthoses and Assistive Devices, 5th ed. Philadelphia, 2019, p. 2-6. DOI: 10.1016/B978-0-323-48323-0.00001-9

[2] Bowers DM, Chui KK. Neurological and Neuromuscular Disease Implications for Orthotic Use. In: Orthotics and Prosthetics in Rehabilitation. 4th ed. 2020. p. 259-293. DOI: 10.1016/B978-0-323-60913-5.00010-6

[3] Lunsford TR, Contoyannis B. Materials Science. In: Atlas of Orthoses and Assistive Devices. 5th ed. Philadelphia. 2019. p. 7-41, DOI: 10.1016/B978-0-323-48323-0.00002-0

[4] Bettoni E, Ferriero G, Bakhsh H, Bravini E, Massazza G, Franchignoni F. A systematic review of questionnaires to assess patient satisfaction with limb orthoses. Prosthetics and orthotics international, 40(2), p. 158-169. DOI: 10.1177/0309364614556836

[5] Supan TJ. Principles of Fabrication. In: Atlas of Orthoses and Assistive Devices. 5th ed. Philadelphia. 2019. p. 42-48. DOI: 10.1016/B978-0-323-48323-0.00003-2

[6] Gibson I, Rosen DW, Stucker B: Additive Manufacturing Technologies. Springer. New York. 2010. 459 p. DOI: 10.1007/978-1-4419-1120-9

[7] Loughborough University: About additive manufacturing [Interne]. 2012. Available from: http://www.lboro.ac.uk/research/amrg/about/the7categoriesofadditivemanufacturing/

[8] International Organization for Standardization: Additive manufacturing [Interne]. Available at: https://www.iso.org/obp/ui/#iso:std:iso-astm:52900:dis:ed-2:v1:en

[9] The new face of biomedical engineering [Interne]. 2016. Available at: https://www.elsevier.com/connect/the-new-face-of-biomedical-engineering

[10] Jorge M. Orthotics and Prosthetics in Rehabilitation: Multidisciplinary Approach. In: Orthotics and Prosthetics in Rehabilitation. 4th ed. 2020. p. 2-13. DOI: 10.1016/B978-0-323-60913-5.00001-5

[11] Zivcak J, Michalikova M, Bednarcikova L. Individual upper limb orthotics. 1st ed. Kosice: Grafotlac; 2016. 179 p.

[12] International Organization for Standardization: Additive manufacturing [Interne]. Available at: https://www.iso.org/obp/ui/#iso:std:iso-astm:52900:ed-1:v1:en

[13] Mohammed MI, Pearse F. Design and additive manufacturing of a patient specific polymer thumb splint concept. In: Solid Freeform Fabrication 2018: Proceedings of the 29th Annual International Solid Freeform Fabrication Symposium – An Additive Manufacturing Conference. November 2018.

[14] Buonamici F, Furfer R, Governi L, Lazzeri S, McGreevy KS, Servi M, Talanti E, Uccheddu F, Volpe Y. A practical methodology for computer-aided design of custom 3D printable casts for wrist fractures. The Visual Computer, 36, p. 375-390. DOI: https: 10.1007/s00371-018-01624-z

[15] Barios-Muriel JB, Romero-Sanchez F, Alonso-Sanchez FJ, Salgado DR. Advances in orthotic and prosthetic manufacturing: a technology review. Materials, 2020, 13, p. 295. DOI: 10.3390/ma13020295

[16] Fitzpatrick A, Mohammed M, Collins P, Gibson I. Design optimization of a thermoplastic splint. In: Solid Freeform Fabrication 2017: Proceedings

of the 28th Annual International: Solid Freeform Fabrication Symposium – An Additive Manufacturing Conference. 2017.

[17] Chen YJ, Lin H, Zhang X, Huang W, Shi L, Wang D. Application of 3D-printed and patient-specific cast for the treatment of distal radius fractures: initial experience. 3D printing in medicine, 2017, 3(11), p. 1-9. DOI: 10.1186/s41205-017-0019-y

[18] Li J, Tanaka H. Rapid customization system for 3D-printed splint using programmable modeling technique – a practical approach. 3D printing in medicine, 2018, 4(5), p. 1-21. DOI: 10.1186/s41205-018-0027-6

[19] Fernandez-Vincent M, Chust AE, Conejero A. Low cost fabrication approach for thumb orthoses. Rapid prototyping journal, October 2017, 23(6), p. 1020-1031. DOI: doi.org/10.1108/RPJ-12-2015-0187

[20] Redaelli DF, Abbate V, Storm FA, Ronca A, Sorrentino A, De Capitani C, Biffi E, Ambrosio L, Colombo G, Fraschini P. 3D printing orthopedic scoliosis braces: a test comparing FDM with thermoforming. In: The International Journal of Advanced Manufacturing Technology. 2020:111:1707-1720. DOI: 10.1007/s00170-020-06181-1

[21] Hale, L., Linley, E. & Kalaskar, D.M. A digital workflow for design and fabrication of bespoke orthoses using 3D scanning and 3D printing, a patient-based case study. Scientific reports, 2020, 10, p. 7028. DOI: 10.1038/s41598-020-63937-1

[22] Stefanovic B, Michalikova M, Bednarcikova L, Trebunova M, Hudak R. Arm and Forearm Scanning Methodology for the Development of an Orthotic Device for Tetraplegic Patients. In: Proceedings of 3DBODY.TECH 2020 - 11th International Conference and Expo on 3D Body Scanning and Processing Technologies. 17-18 November 2020. Online/Virtual

Chapter 7

# Orthoses in Conservative Management of Cerebral Palsy and Rehabilitation

*Akshay Kumar and Vinita*


## Abstract

Cerebral palsy is the developmental and postural disorder that combines a group of conditions/disease (neuromuscular), occurs in the developing fetal or infant brain, affects movement and intelligence that are ascribed to non-progressive disturbances. Orthotics is the branch of modern health science and rehabilitation that deals with assessment, prescription, fabrication, fitment, and purposeful gait training to the individual who needs orthosis for optimal independence. Orthoses are external devices that applied to increase function, prevent contracture and deformity, maintain the limbs in a functional position, stabilize the segments of the body, support the weak muscle and its functions, increase motor control, reduce spasticity, protect the limbs, and body segments in the postoperative condition.


**Keywords:** orthosis, orthotics, cerebral palsy, rehabilitation, conservative management

## 1. Introduction

Cerebral palsy is the developmental and postural disorder that combines a group of conditions/disease (neuromuscular) that occurs in the developing fetal or infant brain, affecting movement and intelligence that are ascribed to non-progressive disturbances [1]. The prevalence of Cerebral Palsy (CP) all over the world reported a range from 1.5 to 4 per 1000 live births and the average birth prevalence is 2 (approx) per 1000 live births. The rate of prevalence observed varies along with the time and region. Now, the rate of CP is relatively stable. However, prematurity and its complication are still the reason for increased prevalence despite improved neonatal and obstetric care [2].

It is important to mention that the one-size-fits-all approach does not work on the population with cerebral palsy. The fitment must be total contact control over the forefoot, hindfoot and ankle to minimize/optimize the deviation in the planes of the foot. Skeletal alignment is the foundation to the operational success of the orthosis. Loosely fitted orthosis may cause discomfort, piston, skin breakdown and ultimately decreased function [3].

In the old world, the "Corpus Hippocraticum" mentions the first medical description of cerebral palsy, which was written by Hippocrates in his work. Nevertheless, it was emerged in the 19th century by William John Little; thus, Little was the first personality to intensely engage cerebral palsy. Two more stalwarts



IntechOpen

William Osler and Sigmund Freud added historical hallmarks to cerebral palsy at the end of the $19^{th}$century. Since then the significant development has been done in the field of cerebral palsy [4]. William Little argued for the earliest possible diagnosis and intervention in the early stages [5].

The environmental access and daily activities in children with CP are restricted due to the development of secondary complications. However, orthoses play an important role in managing and maintaining posture and balance. The purpose of orthotic treatment is to assist function and gait through correction, prevention and providing the base of support [6]. Orthotics is the branch of modern health science and rehabilitation science that deals with assessment, prescription, fabrication, fitment, and purposeful gait training to the individual who needs orthosis for optimal independence [7]. Orthosis is used to preserve the result of surgical procedures during rehabilitation and prevent reoccurrence with growth. The clinician's poor prescription may lead to rejection of the device, complication to the child and psychological compromise to the family [8]. Ankle Foot Orthosis (AFOs) are used frequently in CP to improve function and prevent contractures and have been found to improve walking speed and energy cost [9]. The hinged AFOs results favor the orthotic implication to the CP child by reducing oxygen demand and ventilator cost [10]. The gait laboratory research suggests that there is an indirect effect of orthosis on the joints of limbs and negative effects can be optimized by the appropriate intervention of the orthosis [11].

## 2. Risk factors

Children's risk of being born/identified with cerebral palsy may increase due to some medical condition that happens during pregnancy, delivery and post-delivery. These may be categorized as follows:

### 2.1 Congenital cerebral palsy

This happens before or during birth, damages the brain. In many cases the specific causes are unknown and 80–90% of cases generally found are of congenital cerebral palsy. Some causes increase the chance of a child developing cerebral palsy. Although, it is clear/important that having a risk factor does not confirm that child will have cerebral palsy. Risk factors for Congenital CP areas:

- Low birth weight
- Premature birth
- Multiple births
- Assisted reproductive technology (ART) infertility treatments
- Infections during pregnancy
- Jaundice and kernicterus
- Medical conditions of the mother
- Birth complications

- Blood type incompatibility between mother and child
- Exposure to toxic substances
- Breech presentation
- Small for gestational age

### 2.2 Acquired cerebral palsy

Nearly 10% of diagnosed cases of cerebral palsy in children are considered to be of acquired cerebral palsy caused by damage that occurred in the brain, post-birth. It is accompanied by infection or head injury. The risk factors for acquired cerebral palsy are:

- Preterm or low birth weight
- Brain infections
- Injury
- Infancy
- Not getting certain vaccinations

## 3. Classification

Cerebral Palsy causes functional limitations that lead to disorders of motor and postural development ascribed to non-progressive disorders that happen in fetal development or the child's brain [12]. It has been classified mainly into three categories viz. Physiological, Topographical and Functional classification system, includes Gross Motor Function Classification System (GMFCS), the Manual Ability Classification System (MACS), the Communication Function Classification System (CFCS), and the Eating and Drinking Ability Classification System (EDACS) which are complementary to each other.

### 3.1 Physiological classification of cerebral palsy

I. Spastic—Increased muscle tone in one or more limbs is the primary characteristic. Spastic cerebral palsy is the most common among CP children. It can be unilateral, bilateral, quadrilateral, or hemiplegic [13].

II. Athetotic—It is characterized by the involuntary movement of the affected child and can be recognized in the early days. Hammond described it in 1870 [14].

III. Rigidity

IV. Ataxic

V. Tremor

VI. Atonic

VII. Mixed

VIII. Unclassified [15]

### 3.2 Anatomical/topographical classification (according to the motor deficit) of cerebral palsy

- Hemiplegia—A condition that causes paralysis of half of the body leads to weakness and lack of muscle control.
- Paraplegia—It is motor or sensory impairment that causes loss of function and control over lower limbs or other two limbs.
- Tetraplegia—It is the partial or complete loss of all 4 limbs. Also, known as quadriplegia.
- Triplegia—It's a condition of lack of control or paralysis of three limbs.
- Monoplegia—There is a lack of control of one limb.

Paraplegia is the commonest one followed by hemiplegia and tetraplegia stands third [16].

### 3.3 Functional classification system for cerebral palsy

The functional classification system is categorized into four types which are as follow;

#### *3.3.1 Gross motor function classification system (GMFCS)*

It is the most recognized and established functional classification for Cerebral Palsy. It narrates the gross motor function of the children with cerebral palsy based on an ordinal five-step classification system. GMFCS considers the developmental milestones according to child's age up to 18 years.

*GMFC level I:* Individuals able to walk without limitations.

- Less than 2 years can crawl on knees and hands, pull to stand, and are able to attain independent walking between 18 months to 2 years.
- Between 2 to 4 years of a child are able to sit properly and started sitting to standing transition independently.
- Between 4 and 6 years, the individual should able to walk independently indoors and outdoors, start to run and jump, and climbing stairs.
- Between age 6–12 years, they may develop skills and abilities to walk up and down the curbs, walk community distances.
- Between 12 and 18 individuals in GMFCS I show the capability as of aged 6–12 years old.

*GMFC level II:* Individuals walk with limited endurance and balance with the help of orthoses or assistive devices.

- Before age of 2 children may need body support to sit or stand.
- Between 2 and 4 years, GMFCS II level child may start sitting without support and walk with device support.
- Between 4 and 6 years, they can shift into and out of standing without assistance. Walk indoors without the support and climb up and down the stairs with a railing. However, they cannot jump or run.
- Between 6 and 12 years, children are able to walk on all terrains with certain limitations and need assistive devices or wheeled mobility for long distances.
- Between 12 and 18 years show the same features as of age 6–12 and devices may be required for more safety and support.

*GMFC level III:* Children categorized under GMFC III can walk indoors with the help of assistive devices. However, community mobility needs wheeled devices.

- Below 2 years, can crawl and roll, if posing in the prone position and sit with device support.
- Between 2 and 4 years, the child can "W" sit on the floor with assistance and may stand and walk with the help of handled mobility devices.
- Between 4 and 6 years, GMFC III level categorized child can sit in a chair with adequate support to achieve some upper limb function. Stairs climbing needs assistance and community activity requires wheeled devices respectively.
- From 6 to 18 years the child's remain need assistance to negotiate the stairs and wheeled mobility is required to perform major ADL (Activity of Daily Living) in the community.

*GMFC level IV:* In this category self-mobility is limited but can sit with appropriate support. Preferable mobility options are manual or motorized devices.

- Within 2 years, the child can control their head and may need support to sit.
- Between 2 and 4 years, the child can sit with and stand with appropriate adaptive devices and reciprocal gait movement is generally absent.
- Between 4 and 6 years, children need assistive devices to control the trunk, and sit and wheeled mobility is ideal for community movement.
- Between 6 and 12 years, the child may walk with assistance and can do floor mobility with crawling and rolling.
- From 12 to 18 years, GMFC IV shows the same features as of 6–12 year old.

*GMFC level V:* Power wheeled mobility is possible for self-mobility.

- Below 2 years cannot control head and trunk and assistance is needed for crawling.
- Between 2 and 4 years, a child needs a manual mobility device for mobility.
- After 4 years, the GMFCS V type needs complete assistance in transfer and mobility.

*3.3.2 Manual ability classification system (MACS)*

It is used in children ages 4 to 18 years, developed by Eliasson et al. in 2006. MACS is used for hand and upper extremities based on a five-point ordinal classification system.

MACS I—Individuals can perform the activities independently with minimal or no limitations in case of heavy/fragile objects.

MACS II—Individuals remain independent in daily activities with slower and decreased performance. They may use different ways to handle the objects and perform the activities.

MACS III—Individuals categorized under MACS III may need support or set-up for the activities. They can perform some activities independently and some activities remain requires assistance to be carried out.

MACS IV—Individuals can not be able to complete the task or activities and depends on adaptive devices and continuous assistance to perform the activities.

MACS V—The individuals categorized in MACS V are unable to handle the objects independently. They depend totally on assistance and can perform simple movement.

*3.3.3 Communication function classification system (CFCS)*

It is a valid measure to assess everyday communication in Cerebral palsy. It is also a five-scale ordinal classification system.

CFCS I—Individuals are "effective sender and receiver with unfamiliar and familiar partners" and they can communicate easily with familiar and unfamiliar partners.

CFCS II—In comparison to CFCS I, they communicate at a slower pace with familiar and unfamiliar partners. But, effective in sending and receiving communication.

CFCS III—Individuals are effective communicators with familiar partners. But, due to decreased intelligibility, they can not communicate effectively with unfamiliar partners.

CFCS IV—They can not communicate regularly to familiar partners. Some may communicate occasionally.

CFCS V—Individuals categorized under CFCS V rarely communicate effectively with familiar partners. They regularly have ineffective communication [17].

## 4. Gait patterns in cerebral palsy

The gait patterns ideally vary as per the limb involvement and orthotic treatments take place [18]. The common gait patterns of cerebral palsy that affect the movement and posture can be classified into the following categories based on the sagittal plane kinematics;

A. Unilateral spastic CP

**B.** Bilateral spastic CP

In 1987 Winters et al. classified the gait pattern in spastic hemiplegia. They classified it into four types based on sagittal plane kinematics, which is widely accepted.

Type I – There is drop foot deformity. In the swing phase ankle goes in plantarflexion (PF) while exhibiting adequate dorsiflexion in the stance phase. Management may be needed is a leaf spring or hinged ankle-foot orthosis (AFO).

Type II – It shows tenacious plantarflexion during the stance and swing phase. It is true equines due to contracture or spasticity of gastro-soleus muscles. Further, it can be classified into equinus with the knee in neutral and hip extension, and equines with the knee in recurvatum and hip extension.

Type III – Quadriceps/or hamstring weakness results in reduced knee extension and leads to stiff knee gait during the swing phase. In addition to that, gastro-soleus spasticity causes impaired dorsiflexion in the swing phase.

Type IV – It is characterized by ankle plantarflexion, knee contracture/or restricted knee and hip internal rotation and adduction with limited flexion and extension [19–21].

In Bilateral Spastic CP four main groups were identified based on the ankle, knee, hip, and pelvis kinematics in the sagittal plane proposed by Rodda and Graham [22, 23]. The contractures in one and more joints, imbalance muscle action and muscle spasticity cause gait difficulty in CP. As per evidence observed, mainly four types of gait deformity of the knee have been identified. These are jump knee, crouch knee, stiff knee, and recurvatum knee. The most frequent gait abnormalities occur in the sagittal plane [23].

### 4.1 Gait with equinus foot

Caused by Gastrosoleus spasticity and added recurvatum force the entire foot on toes tip. An orthotic device with 90-degree ankle dorsiflexion, knee extension can be used during the day and night hours post-surgery only.

### 4.2 Jump gait

Children with jump gait show the characteristic of equinus foot, genu flexum, and coxaflecta. Apart from gastrosoleous the spasticity of hamstring and psoas is common in such gait patterns. An orthosis may play an important role in conservative management.

### 4.3 Gait with apparent equinus

Patients show excessive flexion in the knee and hip which leads equinus gait. However, a normal range of dorsiflexion at the ankle is found.

### 4.4 Crouch gait

It is diagnosed by excessive dorsiflexion at the ankle and excessive flexion of the knee and hip joints. Conservative management in such cases aims to maintain posture, alignment, and balance [16, 24, 25].

## 5. Measures to prevent cerebral palsy

Genetics-related cerebral palsy is quite impossible to prevent, and in many cases, the circumstances of congenital cerebral palsy are not fully known and acknowledged. Hence, very little can be done and preventive measures can be taken pre and post-pregnancy to minimize the risk of developmental delays.

Before pregnancy

- Maintaining and improving the health condition of the mother.
- Proper vaccination before getting pregnant.
- Reducing the chance of multiple pregnancies, if opting for assistive reproductive technology (ATR)

During pregnancy

- Parental care training
- Reduce the risk of infection through maintaining hygiene
- Be in touch with the health care provider
- Maintain healthy pregnancy and take nutritious diet

After baby birth

- Keep the baby safe and healthy
- Check for jaundice in and after release from the hospital
- Proper vaccination is needed
- Take preventive measures to prevent injury [26–28].

## 6. Orthotic management

CP is a "progressive neuromuscular deformity" characterized by static neurological deficit and motor function disorder. An understanding of medical consequences and deformities is essential for appropriate prognosis/diagnosis and conservative treatments. It has been observed that, if left untreated, progressive deterioration and disastrous changes in function and gait pattern arise over time. However, the treatment protocols have been changed drastically during the past 50 years, and the cerebral palsy patient is probable survival in contrast to the general population with appropriate health care and orthotic management [29]. Cerebral Palsy impairments result in difficulty in movement, coordination, and balance. Hence, developing treatment plans in such a complex condition is a challenge to promote the health of the child [30]. To maintain the physical well-being in cerebral palsy, orthoses impart/play an important role. The main aim of orthoses implication is to correct, prevent, provide a base of support, and to improve skills and efficiency in movement and function in the lower limb. However, orthoses manage postural impairment in trunks and upper limbs [31].

### 6.1 Orthotic management of lower limb

The main aim of orthotic management in the lower limb in an individual with cerebral palsy is to "correct/or prevent the deformity, to provide sufficient base of support, to provide skill training, and to improve gait pattern. The implication ultimately results in improved Range of Motion (ROM) and level of function. It also helps in maintaining muscle length to bone growth and minimize the secondary effects of the disability [32]. However, orthoses prescribed to correct or prevent the deformities may force some activity limitations by controlling movement [31].

The kinds of orthosis use in the lower limb of cerebral palsy are-as;

1. Foot orthosis (FO)

   Foot orthosis provides a stable base of support. However, it does not interfere with or corrects the deformity.

2. Supra malleolar orthosis (SMO)

   Supra malleolar orthosis may be used to manage foot deformity. Foot management follows the principles of biomechanics, inhibition and facilitation. These biomechanical principles of supra malleolar orthosis must allow the normal pronation and supination to achieve forward movement and normal elongation of the muscles [32]. Supra malleolar orthosis helps in subtalar alignment and gait pattern improvement in children with cerebral palsy and reduces the intensity of symptoms [33]. The supra malleolar orthosis (SMO) also controls midfoot inversion and increases dorsiflexion at the midfoot during the first part of the swing phase [34].

3. Ankle foot orthosis (AFO)

   The most predominantly used orthosis in the lower limb management of CP is AFO. It is used to improve gait patterns, promote stance phase stability, ease swing phase clearance, and limit the contracture of the muscles [35].

4. Floor reaction orthosis (FRO)

   This orthosis is widely used if the child is having crouch gait patterns, which indicate ankle dorsiflexion with increased knee and hip flexion. FROs are also improved postural balance and support the muscles to develop the ability to control the body's Centre of Mass (COM). FROs help in altering the Ground Reaction Forces (GRF) in the sagittal plane and promote external knee extension. Also, it limits the ankle dorsiflexion [36].

5. Knee ankle foot orthosis (KAFO)

   In cerebral palsy Knee Ankle Foot Orthosis (KAFO) is used to maintain posture in standing and during gait training [37]. It is also used to prevent the ankle-foot range of motion in spastic cerebral palsy (SCP) cases [38] and presumed to reduce ankle dorsiflexion ROM at maximum knee extension when applied to six or more than six hours by reducing the muscle-tendon complex stiffness [39].

### 6.2 Upper limb orthotic management

For an Orthotist, management of spasticity, deformity and contractures in the upper extremity are challenging tasks, as the treatment modalities, intervention and objectives differ according to each child [40]. To maintain the joint's position, the static splint is designed and used to stabilize the joints and restrict further deformity. It has shown positive effect if used for a long time. However, prolonged use may cause muscle atrophy and a decrease in muscle function [41]. In comparison, the dynamic splints allow a larger range of motion against resistance and prevent contracture and deformity [42]. Clinicians may use casting of the upper extremity to decrease the tone and improve ROM and increase the muscle length [43]. The opponens hand splint, the hand sandwich, and the Australian splint are used frequently to manage the contracture and deformity. Also, elbow and shoulder orthosis have evidence of correcting flexion and rotation of the elbow and arm [44].

### 6.3 Trunk orthotic management

In general cerebral palsy children do not born with any form of spinal deformity and such things appear with increasing body weight and age. Later on, this may cause respiratory dysfunction and loss of survival [45]. Postural alignment is the major challenge in cerebral palsy children. Prevalence ranges from 15 to 61% with dominance in male children. Spinal deformity increases with age, non-ambulation, spasticity, and muscle weakness [46]. Though the orthotic goal depends on the child's individual needs, the spinal treatment objective is to improve stability/positioning, promote arm and hand function, improve head control, prevent deformity, and improve overall functioning [47]. Some evidence shows that the use of braces may de-accelerate the deformity curve progression in a CP child, proves the technique of conservative management. However, solid evidence is not yet available that spinal braces minimize the rate of surgery [47–49]. The improvement of sitting control and modification in curve progression is the main objective of the conservative management of spinal deformity in cerebral palsy [50]. The improvement in sitting and postural balances was found satisfactory, and a remarkable spinal correction was observed using a 3-point force system with the placement of lateral pads [48]. The nonoperative stable support promotes an upright posture that reduces pain and frees the upper extremity for functional utilization [51]. Braces like Boston, Charleston, Milwaukee, Rosemberger, Wilmington, etc. might be useful to support the cause [52].

## 7. Discussion

The need for orthotic devices differs among the children with cerebral palsy as the clinical needs vary widely. To optimize the children's motor function and gait a wider range of treatment modalities and interventions are required [53]. The implication of supra malleolar orthosis (SMO) may be suitable for controlling deformities like varus or valgus of the foot. It controls sagittal motion during the swing phase with remarkable mid-foot and forefoot kinematic differences [34]. The AFOs are much helpful in achieving ankle stability that impacts trunk motion and promotes body parts coordination, eliminate flexible spasticity and pathological reflexes [54]. Optimistic results of AFOs intervention are observed on energy expenditure, gait kinetics and spatial–temporal kinematic parameters [54, 55]. However, the user's level of deformity and severity may give varied results in controlling movement, posture and adaptation [56]. The children facing the neuro-biomechanical challenge in controlling knee and hip joints may benefit through the distinct AFOs [57]. A structured interview among the parents of Dynamic Ankle Foot Orthoses (DAFO) users about its efficacy reflects positive effects on postural balance and support in standing and sitting [58]. Also, it allows larger total ankle ROM than solid AFOs [59]. Correction of crouch gait pattern by Floor Reaction Ankle Foot Orthosis (FRAFO) of 17 degrees with a standard deviation of 5 degrees can be achieved. This may align knee and postural balance over a longer period [36, 60]. The higher degree of the knee and hip flexion contracture may be considered as a contraindication to the prescription of FRAFOs; were found to restrict the effectiveness of orthosis in controlling knee extension in midstance [61]. The spinal orthosis may help the individual where surgery is not possible. It reduces the scoliotic progression by limiting the deforming forces on the spine and reduces the need for surgery in some cases. Improved head control and social interaction can be achieved with the help of appropriate spinal orthosis [11]. If we study the upper limb orthotic intervention to the children with cerebral palsy, there is a lack of outcome evidence of treatment modality. It indicates the need for more research with vigorous methods to measure the effect of upper limb orthoses and its reliability [62]. According to the type of orthosis and severity of the condition, the orthosis applied to the children with cerebral palsy affects the gait pattern and postural support distinclty [63].

## 8. Conclusions

The orthotic device is part of the health care treatment in cerebral palsy children and it promotes children in maintaining joint, posture and muscle function. The different orthosis has its importance in optimizing functioning and minimizing complications through a stable base of support, improved gait, and reduces spasticity and fall. It helps in creating an accessible environment among children with cerebral palsy, reduces excess energy expenditure. The advancement in diagnosis procedures, development of scientifically proven orthotic devices to limit the primary and secondary impairments through research is the need of the hour. The transparent research on developed orthotic devices for larger number of CP children may create clear consensus on the efficacy.

## Acknowledgements

The author(s) are grateful to Dr. Roshan Bijlee KN, the Director of Composite Regional Centre for Skill Development, Rehabilitation, and Empowerment of Persons with Disabilities, Kozhikode, Kerala, India for his constant technical support.

## Conflict of interest

No potential conflict of interest was reported by the author(s).

## Author details

Akshay Kumar[1*] and Vinita[2]

1 Department of Prosthetics and Orthotics, Composite Regional Centre for Skill Development, Rehabilitation, and Empowerment of Persons with Disabilities, Kozhikode, Kerala, India

2 Pace Rehabilitation, Research, and Artificial Limb Centre, Kozhikode, Kerala, India

*Address all correspondence to: akshaypoist@gmail.com

## References

[1] Cerebral Palsy. PM&R Knowledge now. 2020. Available from: https://now.aapmr.org/cerebral-palsy/

[2] Stavsky M, Mor O, Mastrolia SA, Greenbaum S, Than NG, Erez O. Cerebral palsy-trends in epidemiology and recent development in prenatal mechanisms of disease, treatment, and prevention. Front. Pediatr. 2017;5:1. Available from: www.frontiersin.org

[3] New approaches to orthotic management in children with cerebral palsy. Braceworks Custom Orthotics. 2021. Available from: https://braceworks.ca/2016/08/30/devices/lower-limbs/afo/new-approaches-to-orthotic-management-in-children-with-cerebral-palsy/#Recent-developments-in-healthcare-for-cerebral-palsy

[4] Panteliadis C, Panteliadis P, Vassilyadi F. Hallmarks in the history of cerebral palsy: From antiquity to mid-20th century. Brain Dev. 2013;35:285-292. Available from: http://www.brainanddevelopment.com/article/S0387760412001179/fulltext

[5] Velde, Morgan, Novak, Tantsis, Badawi. Early diagnosis and classification of cerebral Palsy: An historical perspective and barriers to an early diagnosis. J. Clin. Med. 2019;8:1599.

[6] Morris, Christopher SO. Orthotic Management of Children with cerebral Palsy: Journal of Prosthetics and Orthotics. 2002;150-158. Available from: https://journals.lww.com/jpojournal/Fulltext/2002/12000/Orthotic_Management_of_Children_with_Cerebral.5.aspx

[7] Kumar A. Vinita. Current status of prosthetic and orthotic rehabilitation Services in India: Its issues and challenges. Front. Heal. Informatics 2021;10:55. Available from: http://ijmi.ir/index.php/IJMI/article/view/258

[8] Indications for orthoses to improve gait in children with Ce. Journal of the American Academy of Orthopaedic Surgeons. 2021. Available from: https://journals.lww.com/jaaos/Fulltext/2007/03000/Indications_for_Orthoses_to_Improve_Gait_in.8.aspx

[9] Wingstrand M, Hägglund G, Rodby-Bousquet E. Ankle-foot orthoses in children with cerebral palsy: A cross sectional population based study of 2200 children. BMC Musculoskelet. Disord. 2014;15:327. Available from: http://bmcmusculoskeletdisord.biomedcentral.com/articles/10.1186/1471-2474-15-327

[10] Maltais D, Bar-Or O, Galea V, Pierrynowski M. Use of orthoses lowers the O2 cost of walking in children with spastic cerebral palsy. Med. Sci. Sports Exerc. 2001;320-325.

[11] College W, Morris C, Condie D, Fisk J. Recent Developments in Healthcare for Cerebral Palsy: Implications and Opportunities for Orthotics Report of a Meeting. 2008.

[12] Iara Pfeifer L, Baleroni Rodrigues Silva D, Araújo Rodrigues Funayama C, Lício Santos J. Classification of Cerebral Palsy Association between Gender, Age, Motor Type, Topography and Gross Motor Function. 2009.

[13] O'Shea TM. Diagnosis, treatment, and prevention of cerebral Palsy. Clin. Obstet. Gynecol. 2008;51:816-828. Available from: https://journals.lww.com/00003081-200812000-00019

[14] Foley J. Occasional review the athetoid syndrome. A review of a personal series. Neurosurgery, and Psychiatry 1983;46:289-298. Available from: http://jnnp.bmj.com/

[15] Minear WL. A Classification of Cerebral Palsy. 2021. Available from: https://pediatrics.aappublications.org/content/pediatrics/18/5/841.full.pdf

[16] Dana TUGUI R, Antonescu D, Raluca Tugui D. Maedica. Journal of Clinical Medicine Cerebral Palsy Gait, Clinical Importance. 2013.

[17] Andrea Paulson JVA. Overview of four functional classification systems commonly used in cerebral Palsy. Children 2017;4:30. Available from: https://chrome-extension://dagcmkpagjlhakfdhnbomgmjdpkdklff/enhanced-reader.html?pdf=https%3A%2F%2Fbrxt.mendeley.com%2Fdocument%2Fcontent%2Fa66ca803-847e-3450-a8f3-c47428463516

[18] Armand S, Decoulon G, Bonnefoy-Mazure A. Gait analysis in children with cerebral palsy. EFORT Open Rev. 2016;1:448-460. Available from: http://online.boneandjoint.org.uk/doi/10.1302/2058-5241.1.000052

[19] Winters TF, Gage JR, Hicks R. Gait patterns in spastic hemiplegia in children and young adults. J. Bone Jt. Surg. - Ser. A 1987;69:437-441.

[20] Tsitlakidis S, Horsch A, Schaefer F, Westhauser F, Goetze M, Hagmann S, et al. Gait classification in unilateral cerebral Palsy. J. Clin. Med. 2019;8:1652. Available from: https://pmc/articles/PMC6832635/

[21] Classification of Gait Patterns in Cerebral Palsy. Physiopedia. 2021. Available from: https://www.physio-pedia.com/Classification_of_Gait_Patterns_in_Cerebral_Palsy#cite_ref-Winters_5-0

[22] Rodda J, Graham HK. Classification of gait patterns in spastic hemiplegia and spastic diplegia: A basis for a management algorithm. Eur. J. Neurol. 2001;8:98-108. Available from: http://doi.wiley.com/10.1046/j.1468-1331.2001.00042.x

[23] Sutherland DH, Davids JR. Common gait abnormalities of the knee in cerebral palsy. Clin. Orthop. Relat. Res. 1993;139-147. Available from: http://www.ncbi.nlm.nih.gov/pubmed/8458127

[24] Armand S, Decoulon G, Bonnefoy-Mazure A. Gait analysis in children with cerebral palsy. EFORT Open Rev. 2016;1:448-460. Available from: http://online.boneandjoint.org.uk/doi/10.1302/2058-5241.1.000052

[25] Classification of Gait Patterns in Cerebral Palsy. Physiopedia. 2021. Available from: https://www.physio-pedia.com/Classification_of_Gait_Patterns_in_Cerebral_Palsy

[26] Causes and Risk Factors of Cerebral Palsy. CDC. 2020. Available from: https://www.cdc.gov/ncbddd/cp/causes.html

[27] Nelson KB. Causative Factors in Cerebral Palsy. 2008.

[28] Cerebral Palsy. Hope Through Research. National Institute of Neurological Disorders and Stroke. 2020. Available from: https://www.ninds.nih.gov/Disorders/Patient-Caregiver-Education/Hope-Through-Research/Cerebral-Palsy-Hope-Through-Research#3104_7

[29] KN V. Natural history of cerebral Palsy. In: Cerebral Palsy and Early Stimulation. Jaypee Brothers Medical Publishers (P) Ltd.; 2014. page 164-164. Available from: https://www.jaypeedigital.com/book/9789350903018/chapter/ch12

[30] Surveillance of cerebral palsy in Europe: A collaboration of cerebral palsy surveys and registers. Dev. Med. Child Neurol. 2001;42:816. Available from: http://doi.wiley.com/10.1017/S0012162200001511

[31] Morris C. Orthotic Management of Children with cerebral Palsy. J. Prosthetics Orthot. 2002;14:150-158. Available from: http://journals.lww.com/00008526-200212000-00005

[32] Nference C, Management B. International Society for Prosthetics and Orthotics.

[33] Vadivelan K, Manikandan T, Sivakumar VPR. Effect of orthotic subtalar alignment with Co-activation exercise for alteration in gait endurance in a child with cerebral Palsysingle case study. Int. J. Physiother. 2016;3. Available from: https://www.ijphy.org/index.php/journal/article/view/317

[34] Liu X-C, Embrey D, Tassone C, Klingbeil F, Marquez-Barrientos C, Brandsma B, et al. Foot and ankle joint movements inside orthoses for children with spastic CP. J. Orthop. Res. 2014;32:531-536. Available from: http://doi.wiley.com/10.1002/jor.22567

[35] Stott NS. Cerebral pals. In: Management of Chronic Conditions in the Foot and Lower Leg. Elsevier; 2015. page 214-250.Available from: https://linkinghub.elsevier.com/retrieve/pii/B978070204769500008X

[36] Bahramizadeh M, Mousavi ME, Rassafiani M, Aminian G, Ebrahimi I, Karimlou M, et al. The effect of floor reaction ankle foot orthosis on postural control in children with spastic cerebral palsy. Prosthetics Orthot. Int. 2012;36:71-76. Available from: https://journals.lww.com/00006479-201236010-00009

[37] Kwon SH, Lee BS, Lee HJ, Kim EJ, Lee JA, Yang SP, et al. Energy efficiency and patient satisfaction of gait with knee-ankle-foot orthosis and robot (ReWalk)-assisted gait in patients with spinal cord injury. Ann. Rehabil. Med. 2020;44:131-141. doi: 10.5535/arm.2020.44.2.131

[38] Maas JC, Dallmeijer AJ, Oudshoorn BY, Bolster EAM, Huijing PA, Jaspers RT, et al. Measuring wearing time of knee-ankle-foot orthoses in children with cerebral palsy: Comparison of parent-report and objective measurement. Disabil. Rehabil. 2018;40:398-403. Available from: https://www.tandfonline.com/doi/full/10.1080/09638288.2016.1258434

[39] Maas JC, Dallmeijer AJ, Huijing PA, Brunstrom-Hernandez JE, van Kampen PJ, Jaspers RT, et al. Splint: The efficacy of orthotic management in rest to prevent equinus in children with cerebral palsy, a randomised controlled trial. BMC Pediatr. 2012;12:38. Available from: https://bmcpediatr.biomedcentral.com/articles/10.1186/1471-2431-12-38

[40] Chin TYP, Duncan JA, Johnstone BR, Kerr Graham H. Management of the upper limb in cerebral palsy. J. Pediatr. Orthop. B 2005;14:389-404. Available from: http://journals.lww.com/01202412-200511000-00001

[41] Upper Limb Orthotics/Orthotic Intervention for Children with Cerebral Palsy, Wikiversity. 2021. Available from: https://en.wikiversity.org/wiki/Upper_Limb_Orthotics/Orthotic_Intervention_for_Children_with_Cerebral_Palsy

[42] Burtner PA, Poole JL, Torres T, Medora AM, Abeyta R, Keene J, et al. Effect of wrist hand splints on grip, pinch, manual dexterity, and muscle activation in children with spastic hemiplegia: A preliminary study. J. Hand Ther. 2008;21:36-43. Available from: https://linkinghub.elsevier.com/retrieve/pii/S089411300700155X

[43] Lannin NA, Novak I, Cusick A. A systematic review of upper extremity casting for children and adults with central nervous system motor disorders. Clin. Rehabil. 2007;21:963-976.

Available from: http://journals.sagepub.com/doi/10.1177/0269215507079141

[44] Stamp WG. Bracing in Cerebral Palsy.

[45] SATO H. Postural deformity in children with cerebral palsy: Why it occurs and how is it managed. Phys. Ther. Res. 2020;23:8-14. Available from: https://www.jstage.jst.go.jp/article/ptr/23/1/23_R0008/_article

[46] Morrell DS, Pearson JM, Sauser DD. Progressive bone and joint abnormalities of the spine and lower extremities in cerebral Palsy. Radio Graphics 2002;22:257-268. Available from: http://pubs.rsna.org/doi/10.1148/radiographics.22.2.g02mr19257

[47] Pettersson K, Rodby-Bousquet E. Prevalence and goal attainment with spinal orthoses for children with cerebral palsy. J. Pediatr. Rehabil. Med. 2019;12:197-203. Available from: https://www.medra.org/servlet/aliasResolver?alias=iospress&doi=10.3233/PRM-180596

[48] Terjesen T, Lange JE, Steen H. Treatment of scoliosis with spinal bracing in quadriplegic cerebral palsy. Dev. Med. Child Neurol. 2000;42:S0012162200000840. Available from: http://doi.wiley.com/10.1017/S0012162200000840

[49] James WV. Spinal bracing for children with atonic cerebral palsy

[50] Cloake T, Gardner A. The management of scoliosis in children with cerebral palsy: A review. J. Spine Surg. 2016;2:299-309. Available from: http://jss.osspress.com/article/view/3684/4361

[51] Howard JJ, Sees JP, Shrader; M Wade. Current Concept Review Management of Spinal Deformity in Cerebral Palsy. 2019. Available from: www.jposna.org

[52] Zaina F, De Mauroy JC, Grivas T, Hresko MT, Kotwizki T, Maruyama T, et al. Bracing for scoliosis in 2014: State of the art. Eur. J. Phys. Rehabil. Med. 2014;50:93-110. Available from: http://www.ncbi.nlm.nih.gov/pubmed/24622051

[53] Degelaen M. Effect of ankle–foot orthoses on motor performance in cerebral palsy. Dev. Med. Child Neurol. 2018;dmcn.14069. Available from: https://onlinelibrary.wiley.com/doi/abs/10.1111/dmcn.14069

[54] Degelaen M, Leurs F, De Borre L, Kerckhofs E, De Meirleir L, Cheron G, et al. Effect of ankle-foot orthoses on gait in typically developing children: Developmental trend in segmental coordination. J. Pediatr. Rehabil. Med. 2010;3:163-170. Available from: https://www.medra.org/servlet/aliasResolver?alias=iospress&doi=10.3233/PRM-2010-0125

[55] Sukal-Moulton T, de Campos AC, Alter KE, Huppert TJ, Damiano DL. Relationship between sensorimotor cortical activation as assessed by functional near infrared spectroscopy and lower extremity motor coordination in bilateral cerebral palsy. Neuro Image Clin. 2018;20:275-285. Available from: https://linkinghub.elsevier.com/retrieve/pii/S2213158218302353

[56] Aboutorabi A, Arazpour M, Ahmadi Bani M, Saeedi H, Head JS. Efficacy of ankle foot orthoses types on walking in children with cerebral palsy: A systematic review. Ann. Phys. Rehabil. Med. 2017;60:393-402. Available from: https://linkinghub.elsevier.com/retrieve/pii/S1877065717300799

[57] Morris C, Bowers R, Ross K, Stevens P, Phillips D. Orthotic management of cerebral palsy: Recommendations from a consensus conference. Neuro Rehabilitation 2011;28:37-46. Available from: www.ispoint.org.

[58] Bjornson K, Zhou C, Fatone S, Orendurff M, Stevenson R, Rashid S. The effect of ankle-foot orthoses on community-based walking in cerebral Palsy. Pediatr. Phys. Ther. 2016;28:179-186. Available from: https://journals.lww.com/00001577-201628020-00009

[59] Lam WK, Leong JCY, Li YH, Hu Y, Lu WW. Biomechanical and electromyographic evaluation of ankle foot orthosis and dynamic ankle foot orthosis in spastic cerebral palsy. Gait Posture 2005;22:189-197. Available from: https://linkinghub.elsevier.com/retrieve/pii/S0966636204001663

[60] Böhm H, Matthias H, Braatz F, Döderlein L. Effect of floor reaction ankle–foot orthosis on crouch gait in patients with cerebral palsy. Prosthetics Orthot. Int. 2018;42:245-253. Available from: https://journals.lww.com/00006479-201842030-00001

[61] Rogozinski BM, Davids JR, Davis RB, Jameson GG, Blackhurst DW. The efficacy of the floor-reaction ankle-foot orthosis in children with cerebral Palsy. J. Bone Jt. Surgery-America, 2009;91:2440-2447. Available from: http://journals.lww.com/00004623-200910000-00017

[62] Garbellini S, Robert Y, Randall M, Elliott C, Imms C. Rationale for prescription, and effectiveness of, upper limb orthotic intervention for children with cerebral palsy: A systematic review. Disabil. Rehabil. 2018;40:1361-1371. Available from: https://www.tandfonline.com/doi/full/10.1080/09638288.2017.1297498

[63] Kumar A. A prospective evaluation of orthotic device implication on the lower limb in children with cerebral palsy original scientific paper. Hum. Res. Rehabil. 2021;11:12-16.

Chapter 8

# Satisfaction with Orthopedic Treatments

*Cristina Gonzalez-Martin, Sonia Pertega-Diaz, Rocio Seijo-Bestilleiro and Maria Teresa Garcia-Rodriguez*

## Abstract

To determine the effectiveness and satisfaction with orthopodologic treatments in users of the University Clinic of podiatry at the University of A Coruña, according to various parameters. After approval from the ethics committee of the University of A Coruña, an observational retrospective study (n = 125). We analyzed the effectiveness and satisfaction with the orthopodologic treatments depending on the reason for consultation, diagnosis, treatment and goals of treatment. We performed a descriptive analysis of all variables collected. The most frequent reason for consultation was for pain of the hindfoot (58.2%).The most frequent diagnosis was plantar fasciitis, followed by metatarsalgia (29.7% vs. 18.6%). The orthotic treatment corrective was the most used (68.5%) with pronation control (52.3%). The majority of patients reported improvement in pain, and a high degree of satisfaction with the treatment used. The profile of the patient who consults the Podiatry clinic for a orthopodologic treatment is that of a man over the age of 50, who consulted for pain of the hindfoot. The most frequent diagnosis is plantar fasciitis and the treatment carried out the corrective for pronation control. The majority of patients used the brace between 4 and 8 hours a day, with a high satisfaction with the treatment and improvement in the evolution of the pain. The degree of satisfaction was significantly associated with age, younger patients more satisfied. The improvement of pain was significantly associated with age, younger patients who show improvement.

**Keywords:** foot orthosis, orthopedics, orthotic device, patient satisfaction

## 1. Introduction

Podiatry has evolved very quickly in recent years; much progress has been made in: posturology, adapted and individualized plantar orthoses of minimal dimensions, and all with a single purpose, to restore an optimal balance [1].

The realization of customized foot supports has been suffering a constant evolution, although it has not always been accompanied by scientific criteria, but rather by clinical experiences.

Currently, orthopedic treatments are highly demanded by patients and have a high prescription rate in the pathology of the adult foot, whether metatarsalgia (forefoot pain) or talalgia (back pain). In the adult, foot pain, whether due to inflammatory or mechanical causes, is very frequent and results in numerous sick leave and social disturbances [2]. Up to 10% of the population may have pain in the foot, either later or earlier in their lives [3].



IntechOpen

In the adult, the pain of the feet, either of mechanical or inflammatory origin, is very frequent and is the cause of numerous sick leave and social upheavals.

There are numerous studies found in the literature that evaluate the efficacy of plantar orthoses, but all are focused on certain pathologies or alterations, most of these studies are focused on treating very specific alterations of the foot [4–7].

The University Clinic of Podiatry (CUP) of the University of Coruña (UDC), has been providing podiatric service to a large number of patients of all types for more than 10 years, among which the vast majority have multiple pathologies that need conservative treatment par excellence, the plantar orthosis. During the years in which this type of treatment has been carried out, the satisfaction of the patients with the same or the degree of pain improvement has not been evaluated, which is why there is a need to know the satisfaction with the plantar orthosis and the evolution of the main ailment of each patient.

The performance of this study may be justified due to:

The University Podiatry Clinic (CUP) of the Universidade da Coruña (UDC) has been providing podiatric service to a large number of patients of all kinds for more than 10 years, among which the vast majority have multiple pathologies that need conservative treatment due to excellence, the plantar orthosis. During the years in which this type of treatment has been carried out, patients' satisfaction with it and the degree of pain improvement have not been evaluated; therefore the need arises to know the satisfaction with the plantar orthosis and the evolution of the main ailment of each patient. Due to the lack of scientific evidence on the efficacy of orthotic treatments in general, the need has arisen to carry out this study, which aims to make known the estimated reality of the state of the patients we treat, to know their satisfaction with the prescribed treatment and if the same, it has been useful in the disappearance of the pain manifested at the beginning of the consultation.

With the aim of determining the effectiveness and satisfaction with orthopodological treatments in users of the University Clinic of Podiatry (CUP) of the University of Coruña, this study is carried out.

## 2. Methods

An observational retrospective follow-up study was carried out in the university podiatric clinic (CUP) of the University of Coruña (UDC), located in the Naval Hospital of Ferrol (A Coruña). Those patients who came for the first time to the orthopedic service of the University Clinic of Podiatry in the period between September and December 2017 and who gave their written consent to the data collected in the medical history could be used were included in the study for research purposes.

Included in this study were: Patients who attended the orthopodology service of the University Podiatry Clinic of the University of La Coruña for the first time in 2017. Patients who gave their written consent that the data collected in the history can be used for research purposes.

Exclusion criteria: The following were excluded from the study: Patients who did not undergo any orthopedic treatment. Patients whose medical records show that they did not give their written consent that the data collected in the record can be used for research purposes.

We included 125 patients who met the inclusion and exclusion criteria. This sample size allows us to know the effectiveness of the treatment and patient satisfaction with an accuracy of ±8.8% and 95% safety.

The following sociodemographic and clinical variables were studied from each clinical history:

Sociodemographic variables: Age, sex.

Anthropometric variables: Weight, height, body mass index.

Clinical variables: Reason for consultation: forefoot pain, hindfoot pain.

Diagnosis: plantar fasciitis, calcaneal spur, metatarsalgia, flat/pronged foot, first radius insufficiency, others.

Treatment: accommodative plantar orthosis, corrective/functional plantar orthosis.

Treatment objectives: supination control, pronation control, support damping, selectively discharging, compensating for differences (**Figure 1**).

Evaluation of the treatment: In the university clinic of Podiatry of the University of La Coruña, the patients, once the orthopedic treatment has been performed and delivered, the following revisions are made: revision to the month, to the 3 and to the 6 months, and in them it is evaluated: The degree of use of the treatment (it is not used, if it is used and how long), the satisfaction with the applied treatment (little, enough or very satisfied) and the evolution of the main ailment (worsens, without difference, improves slightly or notably).

The effectiveness of the treatment was evaluated by the evolution of the main ailment, according to the self-reported by the patient. Satisfaction with the treatment applied was also recorded according to what was recorded in the clinical history.

The study is authorized by the UDC ethics committee (EC 05/2016). All patients included in the study have previously given their consent for the use of their medical history for research purposes.

### 2.1 Statistic analysis

A descriptive analysis of all the variables collected was carried out.

The degree of use of treatment, the satisfaction with it and the evolution of pain were analyzed at month, at 3 months and at 6 months. To do this, tests were used for paired data, using the Student t test or the Wilcoxon signed rank test for numerical variables and the McNemar test for qualitative variables.

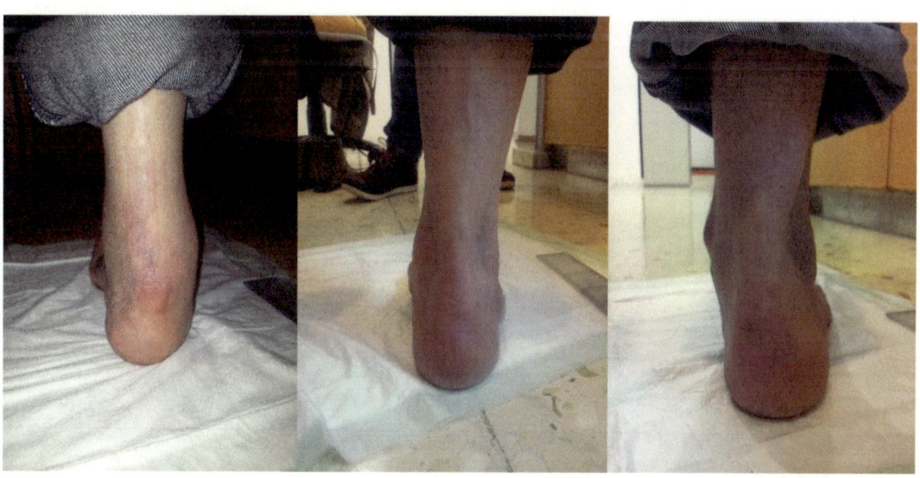

**Figure 1.**
*Rearfoot control.*

The variables related to the effectiveness and satisfaction with the applied treatment were also analyzed. To do this, we used the Student t-test or the Mann–Whitney test for numerical data and the chi-square test or Fisher's exact test for the comparison of percentages. The correlation between quantitative parameters was performed with Spearman's rho correlation coefficient. The normality of the variables was determined by the Kolmogorov–Smirnov test.

## 3. Results

Of the 125 patients included in the study, there was a predominance of males versus females (54.4% vs. 45.6%), with a mean age of 46.0 ± 19.2 years. The body mass index was 28.0 ± 6.2 kg/m$^2$, with a median of 27 and a range of 13.8 to 45.3 kg/m$^2$.

| | n | % | Mean(SD) | Median | Min-Max |
|---|---|---|---|---|---|
| **Age (years)** | 125 | 100% | 46 (19.2) | 51 | 2–81 |
| **Sex** | 125 | 100% | | | |
| Man | 68 | 54.4% | | | |
| Woman | 57 | 45.6% | | | |
| **Weight (kg)** | 105 | | 74.9(19.49 | 73 | 11–132.4 |
| **Size (cm)** | 103 | | 164.1(12.6) | 165 | 126–193 |
| **BMI (kg/m2)** | 103 | | 28(6.2) | 27 | 13.8–45.3 |
| **Reason for consultation** | 110 | | | | |
| Back pain | 64 | 58.2% | | | |
| Forefoot pain | 46 | 41.8% | | | |
| **Diagnosis** | 118 | | | | |
| Fasciitis | 35 | 29.7% | | | |
| Spur calcaneal | 2 | 1.7% | | | |
| Metatarsalgia | 22 | 18.6% | | | |
| Flatfoot | 15 | 12.7% | | | |
| Insufficiency first radio | 5 | 4.2% | | | |
| Others | 39 | 33.1% | | | |
| **Treatment** | 111 | | | | |
| Accommodative | 35 | 31.5% | | | |
| Corrective | 76 | 68.5% | | | |
| **Treatment objectives** | 111 | | | | |
| Pronation control | 58 | 52.3% | | | |
| Supination control | 13 | 11.7% | | | |
| Cushion props | 21 | 18.9% | | | |
| Download supports | 15 | 13.5% | | | |
| Compensate differences | 4 | 3.6% | | | |

*BMI: body mass index.*

**Table 1.**
*Description of the general characteristics of the patients attended in the study period, reasons for consultation and applied treatment.*

Regarding the reason for consultation, the most frequent was hindfoot pain (58.2%) followed by forefoot pain (41.8%). Regarding the diagnosis, the most frequent was plantar fasciitis (29.7%), followed by metatarsalgia (18.6%). The type of orthotic treatment performed most frequently was the corrective (68.5%), followed by the accommodative (31.5%). In relation to the treatment objectives, the most frequent was the control of pronation (52.3%), followed by the cushioning of supports (18.9%) (**Table 1**).

The degree of use of the orthosis, satisfaction and evolution of pain during the follow-up are shown in **Table 2**. In the majority of patients the degree of use was 4–8 hours in the first month as well as in the third and sixth months (75.9%, 77.8% and 75% respectively). Regarding the satisfaction with the treatment, almost two thirds of the patients treated said they were very satisfied with the treatment that has been performed in the first month as well as in the third and sixth (61.2%, 63% and 50% of the patients respectively). And if we evaluate the evolution of pain it is observed that most of the patients have experienced improvement of their pain (noticeable or slight).

Considering the evaluation that the patients made of the satisfaction with the orthosis and of the evolution of the pain in its first review in the clinic (independently of whether it was at one month, three months or six months after treatment) (**Table 3**). 81.8% of them were quite or very satisfied with the treatment, and they also reported a slight or notable improvement in the pain they experienced.

With reference to age, a statistically significant difference in age was observed between satisfied and unmet patients, with significantly younger patients being satisfied than those with little or no satisfaction (44.9 vs. 57.3 years; p = 0.026).

In turn, patients less satisfied with the treatment showed higher BMI values, although without statistically significant differences (29.4 vs. 27.6, p = 0.132).

| | **1 month** | | **3 months** | | **6 months** | |
|---|---|---|---|---|---|---|
| | n | % | n | % | n | % |
| **Degree of use** | 54 | 100% | 27 | 100% | 28 | 100% |
| Null | 2 | 3.7% | 0 | 0% | 0 | 0% |
| Occasional | 3 | 5.6% | 0 | 0% | 0 | 0% |
| Daily | 8 | 14.8% | 6 | 22.2% | 7 | 25% |
| <4 hours | 0 | 0% | 0 | 0% | 0 | 0% |
| 4–8 hours | 41 | 75,9% | 21 | 77.8% | 21 | 75% |
| **Satisfaction with the orthosis** | 54 | 100% | 27 | 100% | 28 | 100% |
| Nothing satisfied | 4 | 7.4% | 1 | 3.7% | 0 | 0% |
| Little satisfied | 6 | 11.1% | 4 | 14.8% | 5 | 17.9% |
| Pretty satisfied | 11 | 20.4% | 5 | 18.5% | 9 | 32.1% |
| Very satisfied | 33 | 61.2% | 17 | 63% | 14 | 50% |
| **Evolution of pain** | 54 | 100% | 27 | 100% | 28 | 100% |
| Gets worse | 3 | 5.6% | 1 | 3.7% | 0 | 0% |
| Without difference | 8 | 14.8% | 4 | 14.8% | 4 | 14.3% |
| It slightly improves | 12 | 22.2% | 6 | 22.2% | 11 | 39.3% |
| Significantly improves | 31 | 57.4% | 16 | 59.3% | 13 | 46.4% |

**Table 2.**
*Degree of use of the orthosis, satisfaction and evolution of pain during follow-up.*

A greater percentage of satisfaction with the orthosis was observed in men than in women (86.4% vs. 75.8%, $p = 0.232$), as well as in patients who consulted for forefoot pain compared to those who presented pain of hindfoot (89.3% vs. 76.6%, $p = 0.172$), although in none of the cases did the differences reach statistical significance. There were also no differences in the degree of satisfaction according to the established diagnosis, the type of treatment or its objective (**Table 3**).

The evolution of pain self-reported by patients after treatment with the orthosis, according to different variables, is shown in **Table 4**. Patients who report mild or notable improvement are significantly younger (44.8 vs. 57.8 years, $p = 0.018$) and have a lower body mass index (27.5 vs. 29.8 kg/m$^2$; $p = 0.061$), although in this case without reaching statistical significance. Again men report a greater percentage of pain improvement than women (86.4% vs. 75.8%,

| | **Nothing/little satisfied** | | **Quite/ very satisfied** | | |
|---|---|---|---|---|---|
| | **Mean (SD)** | **Median** | **Mean (SD)** | **Median** | **p** |
| **Age(years)** | 57.3 (16.8) | 59.5 | 44.9 (18.8) | 47 | 0.026 |
| **BMI (kg/m$^2$)** | 29.4(5.7) | 31.2 | 27.6 (5.9) | 26.5 | 0.132 |
| | **n** | **%** | **n** | **%** | |
| **Total** | **14** | **18.2%** | **63** | **81.8%** | |
| **Sex** | | | | | 0.232 |
| Man | 6 | 13.6% | 38 | 86.4% | |
| Woman | 8 | 24.2% | 25 | 75.8% | |
| **Reason for consultation** | | | | | 0.172 |
| Back pain | 11 | 23.4% | 36 | 76.6% | |
| Forefoot pain | 3 | 10.7% | 25 | 89.3% | |
| **Diagnosis** | | | | | — |
| Fasciitis | 3 | 13.6% | 19 | 86.4% | |
| Spur calcaneal | 0 | 0% | 2 | 100% | |
| Metatarsalgia | 3 | 23.1% | 10 | 76.9% | |
| Flatfoot | 3 | 25% | 9 | 75% | |
| Insufficiency first radio | 1 | 25% | 3 | 75% | |
| Others | 4 | 16.7% | 20 | 83.3% | |
| **Treatment** | | | | | 0.745 |
| Accommodative | 3 | 13.6% | 19 | 86.4% | |
| Corrective | 11 | 20% | 44 | 80% | |
| **Treatment objectives** | | | | | |
| Pronation control | 9 | 21.4% | 33 | 78.6% | |
| Supination control | 2 | 22.2% | 7 | 77.8% | |
| Cushion | 1 | 9.1% | 10 | 90.9% | |
| Download supports | 2 | 16.7% | 10 | 83.3% | |
| Compensate differences | 0 | 0% | 3 | 100% | |

*BMI: body mass index.*

**Table 3.**
*Analysis of the satisfaction of patients with the treatment at the first visit that come to review the clinic, according to different variables.*

| | Worse/no difference | | Improvement slightly/ noticeably | | |
|---|---|---|---|---|---|
| | **Mean (SD)** | **Median** | **Mean (SD)** | **Median** | **p** |
| **Age (years)** | 57.8 (16.9) | 59.5 | 44.8 (18.7) | 47 | 0.018 |
| **BMI (kg/m2)** | 29.8 (5.38) | 31.2 | 27.5 (5.9) | 26.4 | 0.061 |
| | **n** | **%** | **n** | **%** | |
| **TOTAL** | **14** | **18.2%** | **63** | **81.8%** | |
| **Sex** | | | | | 0.232 |
| Man | 6 | 13.6% | 38 | 86.4% | |
| Woman | 8 | 24.2% | 25 | 75.8% | |
| **Reason for consultation** | | | | | 0.172 |
| Back pain | 11 | 23.4% | 36 | 76.6% | |
| Forefoot pain | 3 | 10.7% | 25 | 89.3% | |
| **Diagnosis** | | | | | |
| Fasciitis | 3 | 13.6% | 19 | 86.4% | |
| Spur calcaneal | 0 | 0% | 2 | 100% | |
| Metatarsalgia | 2 | 15.4% | 11 | 84.6% | |
| Flatfoot | 3 | 25% | 9 | 75% | |
| Insufficiency first radio | 1 | 25% | 3 | 75% | |
| Others | 5 | 20.8% | 19 | 79.2% | |
| **Treatment** | | | | | 0.745 |
| Accommodative | 3 | 13.6% | 19 | 86.4% | |
| Corrective | 11 | 20% | 44 | 80% | |
| **Treatment objectives** | | | | | |
| Pronation control | 9 | 21.4% | 33 | 78.6% | |
| Supination control | 2 | 22.2% | 7 | 77.8% | |
| Cushion | 0 | 0% | 11 | 100% | |
| Download supports | 3 | 25% | 9 | 75% | |
| Compensate differences | 0 | 0% | 3 | 100% | |

*BMI: body mass index.*

**Table 4.**
*Analysis of the evolution of pain with self-reported treatment by patients at the first visit to which they come to review the clinic, according to different variables.*

p = 0.232), as well as patients with forefoot pain compared to those who complain of hindfoot pain (89, 3% vs. 76.6%, p = 0.172), although these differences are not statistically significant. The established diagnosis, the type of treatment applied or the objective of the treatment are not associated with the degree of pain improvement (**Table 4**).

## 4. Discussion

In the present study we have tried to verify that the plantar orthosis is a conservative method of treatment that has been used in patients of all ages, and in multiple foot pathologies. 81.8% of the patients who attend the CUP are satisfied with the treatment main ailment has improved, compared to 18.2% who are not satisfied and their ailment remains the same. Patients who have improved are relatively younger, and with lower BMI.

The effectiveness of the orthoses performed at the University Clinic of Podiatry of the University of La Coruña, has been demonstrated in this study, where in most cases the satisfaction of patients, and the evolution of self-reported pain has improved.

In a review found in the literature, it is shown that in adults with different pathologies such as cavus foot, rheumatoid arthritis (RA), the custom-made foot orthosis reduces the patient's pain [4].

This review focuses only on tailor-made foot orthoses, which are defined in this review as removable, anatomical devices that are placed inside the footwear and are molded or manufactured from a foot print and manufactured according to the specifications prescribed by the doctor, in this case a podiatrist.

Foot pain may be experienced after an injury; overuse in the long term; infection; or systemic diseases that include any foot tissue, including bones, joints, ligaments, muscles, tendons, nerves, skin and nails. Foot pain can be generalized or diagnosed more specifically according to location (eg, heel pain), structure (eg, ligament or tendon damage) or disorder (eg, osteoarthritis) [8].

In another review found [9] carried out in children, the effect of non-surgical treatments for flatfoot is proven and shows that in children with flat feet and juvenile idiopathic arthritis, customized foot orthoses can slightly improve pain and function of the foot. Currently, the evidence from randomized controlled trials is too limited to draw definitive conclusions about the use of nonsurgical interventions for pediatric flatfoot. Future trials of high quality in this field are required. Only limited interventions that are frequently used in practice have been studied and there is much debate about the treatment of symptomatic and asymptomatic flatfoot [9].

We found several studies that speak about the use of plantar orthoses for the flatfoot [10–12] and the results of the studies speak of improvement in plantar pressures, as well as in the control of anomalous movements.

There are numerous studies in the literature that speak about the effects of plantar orthoses, both in the population with previous pathology such as arthritis, osteoarthritis, diabetic population, plantar fasciitis [13–18], as well as in people who practice sports and the effect that orthosis produces in the practice of certain sports practice [15].

For example, in the studies carried out by Hähni M [19] and Munteau S [20], the effectiveness of plantar orthoses in reducing plantar pressures and Achilles tendinopathies is highlighted.

It has been shown in the study by Coheña-Jiménez [7] that treatment with plantar orthoses is effective for plantar fasciitis. There are many studies that show the benefits of orthosis treatment, it would be good to carry out more studies focused on evaluating the efficacy in the treatment of flat feet, cavus for example. It is very difficult to evaluate patient satisfaction in this sense, since in most cases they are evaluated by pain improvement, so it would be good to have other measurement systems in which we could quantify patient satisfaction.

More studies are needed to evaluate satisfaction and effectiveness of the foot orthoses made to measure for the foot, especially to check if in certain pathologies it is possible to reduce pain and overload in the plantar pressures, something that would be very beneficial for the patient.

Selection biases Selection biases may arise from the inclusion and exclusion criteria determined for the execution of the study. In our case, they will also be determined by the patients' decision to participate. To minimize these biases, the results will be compared with those of other similar studies.

Information biases: Information biases arising from how the data were obtained may occur: Variability produced by the type of procedure or test used to carry out the examinations, these biases can be minimized, as far as possible, through the establishment of validated questionnaires, calibrated instruments, training of observers.

Confusion biases Due to the absence of variables in the data collection that should have been taken into account for the realization of this study and that are not included due to ignorance of them. To minimize this bias, a multivariate logistic regression analysis will be performed.

## 5. Conclusions

1. The profile of the patient who consults in the podiatric clinic of the UDC for an orthopodological treatment is a male around 50 years of age, who consults for hindfoot pain. The most frequent diagnosis is that of plantar fasciitis and the orthotic treatment performed the corrective to control pronation.

2. The majority of patients use the orthosis between 4 and 8 hours a day, showing a high satisfaction with the treatment and improvement in the evolution of pain.

3. The degree of satisfaction is significantly associated with age, with younger patients being more satisfied. Greater satisfaction is observed in males, in patients with forefoot pain and lower body mass index, although without significant differences. The degree of satisfaction is not associated with the diagnosis, type and objective of the treatment.

4. The improvement in pain is significantly associated with age, the patients who show improvement with the pain younger. Men, with forefoot pain and lower body mass index, reported a greater degree of improvement, although without significant differences. The improvement of pain is also not associated with the diagnosis, type and objective of the treatment.

## Author details

Cristina Gonzalez-Martin*, Sonia Pertega-Diaz, Rocio Seijo-Bestilleiro and Maria Teresa Garcia-Rodriguez
Rheumatology and Public Health Research Group, Nursing Research and Health Care, Biomedical Research Institute of A Coruña (INIBIC), Complejo Hospitalario Universitario de A Coruña (CHUAC), SERGAS, University of Coruña (UDC), Coruña, Spain

*Address all correspondence to: cristina.gmartin@udc.es

## References

[1] Villenueve P. Tratamiento postural y ortesis podal: ¿mecánica o información? Revista IPP. Revista del Instituto de Posturología y Podoposturología. Año 1, Núm 2(2008). ISSN 1988-8198.

[2] Cohía O, Salinasb F. Ortesis plantares. Rev Esp Reumatol 2003; 30(9):508-513

[3] Vázquez Arcea, M.I. Alcañiz Alberolab, M. Nu-Cornejo Palomaresc, C. Mollad, J. Núñez-Cornejo Piquerb, C. Utilidad de las plantillas conformadas. Rehabilitación (Madrid). 2010; 44 (4):291-297.

[4] Kristanto A, Neubert MS, Gross MT, Puntumetakul R, Kaber DB, Sessomboon W. Effects of corrective insole on leg muscle activation and lower extremity alignment in rice farmers with pronated foot: a preliminary report. Foot (Edinb). 2020 Dec 25;46:101771. doi: 10.1016/j.foot.2020.101771. Epub ahead of print. PMID: 33454606.

[5] Paterson KL, Hinman RS, Metcalf BR, Jones SE, Menz HB, Munteanu SE, Kasza J, Bennell KL. Foot orthoses for first metatarsophalangeal joint osteoarthritis: study protocol for the FORT randomised controlled trial. BMC Musculoskelet Disord. 2020 Dec 10;21(1):830. doi: 10.1186/s12891-020-03809-x. PMID: 33302926; PMCID: PMC7726603.

[6] Hoeffner R, Agergaard AS, Funaro A, Bjerregaard N, Svensson RB, Alkjaer T, Magnusson SP. The influence of an orthopaedic walker boot on forefoot force. Foot (Edinb). 2020 Sep 10;46:101739. doi: 10.1016/j.foot.2020.101739. Epub ahead of print. PMID: 33285492.

[7] Coheña-Jiménez M, Pabón-Carrasco M, Pérez Belloso AJ. Comparison between customised foot orthoses and insole combined with the use of extracorporeal shock wave therapy in plantar fasciitis, medium-term follow-up results: A randomised controlled trial. Clin Rehabil. 2020 Nov 24:269215520976619. doi: 10.1177/0269215520976619. Epub ahead of print. PMID: 33233945.

[8] Hawke Fiona, Burns Joshua, Radford Joel A, du Toit Verona. Ortesis de pie hecha a medida para el tratamiento del dolor de pie (Revisión Cochrane traducida). En: La Biblioteca Cochrane Plus, 2008 Número 4.

[9] Rome K, Ashford R, Evans A. Intervenciones no quirúrgicas para el pie plano pediátrico. Cochrane Database of Systematic Reviews 2012 Issue 11. Art. No.: CD006311. DOI: 10.1002/14651858.CD006311.

[10] Pardos Barrado M. Sala Gutiérrez E. Estudio cinemático del efecto del soporte plantar en la rotación interna de la pierna en un niño con pie plano flexible. Rev Int Ciencias Podológicas. 2009; 3 (1): 15-34.

[11] Bok SK, Lee H, Kim BO, Ahn S, Song Y, Park I. The Effect of Different Foot Orthosis Inverted Angles on Plantar Pressure in Children with Flexible Flatfeet. PLoS One. 2016 Jul 26;11(7):e0159831. doi: 10.1371/journal.pone.0159831. PubMed PMID: 27458719; PubMed Central PMCID: PMC4961415.

[12] Tang SF, Chen CH, Wu CK, Hong WH, Chen KJ, Chen CK. The effects of total contact insole with forefoot medial posting on rearfoot movement and foot pressure distributions in patients with flexible flatfoot. Clin Neurol Neurosurg. 2015 Feb;129 Suppl 1:S8-11. doi: 10.1016/S0303-8467(15)30004-4. PubMed PMID: 25683316.

[13] Chapman GJ, Halstead J, Redmond AC. Comparability of off the shelf foot orthoses in the redistribution of forces in midfoot osteoarthritis patients. Gait Posture. 2016 Sep;49:235-240. doi: 10.1016/j.gaitpost.2016.07.012. PubMed PMID: 27459418; PubMed Central PMCID: PMC5038933.

[14] Heuch L, Streak Gomersall J. Effectiveness of offloading methods in preventing primary diabetic foot ulcers in adults with diabetes: a systematic review. JBI Database System Rev Implement Rep. 2016 Jul;14(7):236-65. doi: 10.11124/JBISRIR-2016-003013. PubMed PMID: 27532798.

[15] Hatton AL, Dixon J, Rome K, Brauer SG, Williams K, Kerr G. The effects of prolonged wear of textured shoe insoles on gait, foot sensation and proprioception in people with multiple sclerosis: study protocol for a randomized controlled trial. Trials. 2016 Apr 21;17(1):208. doi: 10.1186/s13063-016-1337-x. PubMed PMID: 27098452; PubMed Central PMCID: PMC4839159.

[16] Lewis RD, Wright P, McCarthy LH. Orthotics Compared to Conventional Therapy and Other Non-Surgical Treatments for Plantar Fasciitis. J Okla State Med Assoc. 2015 Dec;108(12):596-598. Review. PubMed PMID: 26855444; PubMed Central PMCID: PMC4742336.

[17] Munteau S. Landorf B. Menz H. Cook JL. Pizzari T. Scott L. Efficacy of customised foot orthoses in the treatment of Aquilles tendinopathy: Study protocol for a randomised trial. Journal of foot and ankle research. 2009; 2-27.

[18] Roos E. Engstrom M. Soderberg B. Foot orthoses for the treatment of plantar fascitis. Foot and ankle international. Vol 27 N°8(2006).

[19] Hähni M, Hirschmüller A, Baur H. The effect of foot orthoses with forefoot cushioning or metatarsal pad on forefoot peak plantar pressure in running. J Foot Ankle Res. 2016 Nov 16;9:44. PubMed PMID: 27891180; PubMed Central PMCID: PMC5112690.

[20] Munteau S. Landorf B. Menz H. Cook JL. Pizzari T. Scott L. Efficacy of customised foot orthoses in the treatment of Aquilles tendinopathy: Study protocol for a randomised trial. Journal of foot and ankle research. 2009; 2-27.